ACCESSING the HEALING POWER of the VAGUS NERVE

ACCESSING the HEALING POWER of the VAGUS NERVE

SELF-HELP EXERCISES FOR ANXIETY, DEPRESSION, TRAUMA, AND AUTISM

Stanley Rosenberg

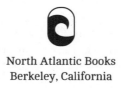

North Atlantic Books
Berkeley, California

Published by
North Atlantic Books
Berkeley, California

Cover art by Jasmine Hromjak. All other illustrations by Sohan Mie Poulsen; © Stanley Rosenberg 2017. Photographs by Tau Bjorn Rosenberg
Cover design by Nicole Hayward
Book design by Suzanne Albertson

Printed in Canada

Accessing the Healing Power of the Vagus Nerve: Self-Help Exercises for Anxiety, Depression, Trauma, and Autism is sponsored and published by the Society for the Study of Native Arts and Sciences (dba North Atlantic Books), an educational nonprofit based in Berkeley, California, that collaborates with partners to develop cross-cultural perspectives, nurture holistic views of art, science, the humanities, and healing, and seed personal and global transformation by publishing work on the relationship of body, spirit, and nature.

North Atlantic Books' publications are available through most bookstores. For further information, visit our website at www.northatlanticbooks.com or call 800-733-3000.

MEDICAL DISCLAIMER: The following information is intended for general information purposes only. Individuals should always see their health care provider before administering any suggestions made in this book. Any application of the material set forth in the following pages is at the reader's discretion and is his or her sole responsibility. The author takes full responsibility for representing and interpreting the ideas related to the Polyvagal Theory. The author's interpretations and representations of the Polyvagal Theory may vary in intent and accuracy from the writings and presentations by Dr. Stephen W. Porges.

Library of Congress Cataloging-in-Publication Data

Rosenberg, Stanley, 1940–
    Accessing the healing power of the vagus nerve : self-help exercises for anxiety,
    depression, trauma, and autism / Stanley Rosenberg.
        pages cm
    ISBN 978-1-62317-024-0 (Trade paperback) — ISBN 978-1-62317-025-7 (Ebook)
    1. Depression, Mental—Alternative treatment. 2. Anxiety—Alternative treatment.
    3. Autism—Alternative treatment. 4. Vagus nerve. 5. Self-care, Health. I. Title.
    RC537.R63844 2016
    616.85'27—dc23   2015028780

6 7 8 9 MARQUIS 23 22 21 20
This book includes recycled material and material from well-managed forests. North Atlantic Books is committed to the protection of our environment. We print on recycled paper whenever possible and partner with printers who strive to use environmentally responsible practices.

To Linda Thorborg

TABLE OF CONTENTS

FOREWORD

I met Stanley in June 2002, when I spoke at the United States Association for Body Psychotherapy Conference in Baltimore. The evening before my talk I received a message from Jim Oschman asking if he and Stanley could attend. Jim explained that I would enjoy meeting Stanley and learning about his work. After my talk, Stanley explained his desire to identify objective measures, such as heart rate variability, that could be used to conduct research to validate the clinical work he was doing.

I was curious and wanted to learn more about his work, his approach, and why he was interested in measurements of vagal function. I mentioned to him that I had spondylolisthesis, a condition in which a vertebra slides forward over the bone below it. He casually responded, "I can fix it." I asked him how long he thought it would take. He said about ten to fifteen seconds! At this point I was trying to figure out what he could do in ten to fifteen seconds. I had assumed, based on his training in Rolfing and craniosacral techniques, that his treatment would require several sessions. Given my history with an orthopedic specialist, I was curious if a somatic therapy could be effective. The suggestion that it could be rehabilitated in a few seconds was outside my worldview.

My diagnosis was based on a slippage in the lower spine at the junction of lumbar and sacral vertebrae. The slippage caused back pain and possibly a progressive deterioration that would lead to surgery. I was diagnosed by an orthopedic surgeon, who imposed on me a fear of surgery to motivate progress in physical therapy. Following my graduation from physical therapy, I went to a sports medicine physician who prescribed a back brace to limit mobility. From this portfolio of health care professionals, I received contradictory instructions; the physicians encouraged me to immobilize the lower back, while the physical therapists encouraged me to move and work on flexibility. By the time I met Stanley, it was not clear to me how to treat my condition to minimize symptoms and avoid surgery.

When Stanley generously offered to "fix it," I welcomed the opportunity. Stanley instructed me to go on my hands and knees, and to relax and keep my spine relatively level. Then, with the fingers from both hands going in opposing directions, he moved the tissue over the vertebrae that had slipped. As he did this, the vertebrae immediately and effortlessly slipped into position. For fifteen years I have used a modification of his procedure to remain pain free.

I understood immediately what he was doing. The physical manipulation, which gently moved the upper levels of tissue, signaled the body to relax. The relaxation was sufficient to reorganize the neural muscular regulation that supported the spine, allowing the vertebra to gently fall into place. Thus Stanley was transmitting signals of safety to the neuromuscular system that enabled the system to immediately shift from a defensive state of contraction, in which it attempted to protect the vulnerability of the lower spine, to a state of safety in which a gentle touch would functionally allow the system to find its natural position.

Stanley's method confirmed that a metaphor of safety is manifest throughout the body and not merely in the social engagement system via the muscles of the face and head, or in the viscera via ventral vagal pathways. In all aspects of the human anatomy, safety is expressed by the down regulation and the constraint of defense. When safety occurs, the structures can retune themselves to support health, growth, and restoration. Functionally, Stanley's work is based on his implicit understanding that when the nervous system is manifest in a state of safety there is a welcoming to touch, which can be used to align bodily structures and optimize autonomic function.

Our first meeting captured Stanley's essence and brilliance. It captured his passionate desire to alleviate pain and suffering. It captured his compassionate approach that supports states of safety through gentle co-regulation. And it captured his intuitive understanding of the integrated systems of the body.

Stanley and I have now been good friends for fifteen years. In multiple visits we have discussed how his manipulations shift autonomic state to promote health, growth, and restoration. As this book conveys, he has brilliantly integrated features of the Polyvagal Theory with features from craniosacral and other somatic therapies. To do this, he artfully extracted the primary principle of the Polyvagal Theory: the structures of the body become welcoming to touch and manipulation when in a state of safety.

According to the Polyvagal Theory, the body, including the neural regulation of skeletal muscle, functions differently when in a state of safety. In the state of safety, ventral vagal pathways coordinate the autonomic nervous system. In this state, the defensive features of the autonomic nervous system are constrained, and the body is welcoming not only to the social engagement behaviors of prosodic vocalizations and facial expressions, but to touch. Underlying Stanley's clinical successes is his ability to connect and co-regulate the client through interactions between the client's social engagement systems, and to convey cues of trust and concern that trigger the beneficial attributes of the ventral vagal circuit in promoting a state of safety through the entire body.

Stanley is not a traditional therapist trained within a discipline. His training crosses disciplines, and his approach is more consistent with the traditions of a healer. Healers enable the body to heal itself, and Stanley functions in this role. He co-regulates his clients, enabling and empowering them to heal through the body's own mechanisms. His interest in the Polyvagal Theory comes from his implicit understanding that when states of safety are manifest in the structures of the body, the body is poised to serve as a platform for healing.

Accessing the Healing Power of the Vagus Nerve is Stanley's personal expression of his insight into and appreciation of the role that vagal pathways play in the healing process by calming the body and enabling the body to welcome touch. By intuitively understanding this integrated process, Stanley has developed a system of manipulations that promote states of safety, allowing the body to retune the nervous system, thus optimizing behavior, mental health, and physiological homeostasis.

As a scientist, I do not experience the world of the therapist. As a therapist, Stanley does not experience the world as a scientist. However, Stanley's gift lies in his ability to implicitly organize information from science and to apply it therapeutically in an intuitive, insightful, and helpful manner. Stanley's contributions as a creative therapist are unique within the complex health care environment. Fortunately, his powerful insights, metaphors, and treatment models are beautifully conveyed and archived in *Accessing the Healing Power of the Vagus Nerve.*

Stephen W. Porges, PhD,
Distinguished University Scientist, Kinsey Institute,
Indiana University, and professor of psychiatry,
University of North Carolina

FOREWORD

There are times in history when need is met with equal brilliance. We are blessed with one of these rare moments. Stanley Rosenberg's *Accessing the Healing Power of the Vagus Nerve* gives the reader tools to navigate and treat some of the most complex of maladies.

Stanley brings forward this new wave of thought with the foundation of his almost half-century of clinical experience, trainings, and teaching. *Accessing the Healing Power of the Vagus Nerve* provides insights into the genesis of physical and emotional conditions, the reasons why they often have not been successfully treated with conventional methods, and effective tools to resolve them.

Our well-being is dependent on a functional and adaptive nervous system. At the heart of our adaptability, especially to stress, is the vagus nerve. This cranial nerve is integrated into our entire physical and neurological matrix. The vagus nerve is central to every aspect of our life. It can provide us with deep relaxation as well as offer immediate response to life-and-death situations. It can be both the cause and the resolution of countless disorders. Additionally, the vagus nerve can provide us with the needed deep personal connection to others and our environment.

I have had the privilege of knowing Stanley for over thirty-five years. I have studied together with him, learned from him, and taught for the Rosenberg Institute. I know of no other practitioner more qualified to bring together all the essential elements that are presented in this book.

Accessing the Healing Power of the Vagus Nerve unlocks the mysteries of chronic disorders. There are many books published that explain these conditions, but none so successfully delves into the underlying basis of how and why these conditions develop.

Whether for therapists, sufferers, or simply readers who wish to learn more about themselves and others, *Accessing the Healing Power of the Vagus Nerve* is a must-read. We owe Stanley Rosenberg a debt of gratitude that he has woven his decades of insight into a fascinating and unforgettable work.

Benjamin Shield, PhD,
author of *Healers on Healing, For the Love of God,*
Handbook for the Soul, and *Handbook for the Heart*

ACKNOWLEDGMENTS

Thanks to Stephen Porges, who formulated the Polyvagal Theory—his teaching and writings opened a world of understanding and have allowed me to help many people in my clinic and to teach other clinicians. He has been a friend for more than a decade and an inspiration in my formulating and writing of this book. He also reviewed an early draft of this manuscript and helped to clarify important points.

Thanks to Alain Gehin, my friend, mentor, and primary teacher in osteopathy and craniosacral therapy for more than twenty-five years. I also extend my gratitude to Professor Pat Coughlin at Geisinger Commonwealth School of Medicine (formerly known as the Commonwealth Medical College), who has been my main teacher of anatomy and physiology and who helped to edit the anatomical references in this text. Linda Thorborg was an inspiration in the development of many aspects of my hands-on techniques and has co-taught optimal-breathing courses with me.

Thanks to Kathy Glass, my developmental editor, who took my chaotic notes and shaped them into this book. I have been living in Denmark and speaking Danish for thirty-five years, and my English language, especially my written language, has suffered. Looking back, I see that Kathy took on a near-impossible task of helping me to formulate my thoughts—and completed it with style. Benjamin Shield and Jacqueline Lapidus also helped me with the editing of early drafts.

Also, thanks to Mary Buckley, Erin Wiegand, and Nina Pick, editors from North Atlantic Books, who helped put my manuscript into its final shape.

Thanks to some of my other teachers, including Jim Oschman, who wrote the book *Energy Medicine;* Tom Myers, author of the book *Anatomy Trains;* my four teachers in tai chi and chi gung: John Chung Li, Ed Young, Professor Cheng Man-Ch'ing, and Hans Finne; my teacher in mindfulness and Vipassana meditation, Joseph Goldstein; my teachers in Rolfing®: Peter Melchior, Peter Schwind, Michael Salveson, and Louis Schultz; and Timothy Dunphy, Ann Parks, and my other teachers in healing, massage, and other body therapies over the years.

Thanks also to my colleagues at the Stanley Rosenberg Institute, as well as all of my students, patients, and my many friends over the years, especially Ira Brind, Benjamin Shield, Anne and Philip Neess, Lise Pagh, Charlotte Soe, Mohammed Al Mallah, Gordon Enevoldson, DeeDee Schmidt Petersen, Trine Rosenberg, and Donna Smith. Thanks to Filip Rankenberg and my other colleagues at Manuvision.

Also, thanks to Sri Sri Ravi Shankar for his interest in our form of craniosacral therapy and for his support over the years.

Thanks to my children, Annatrine, Erik, and Tau; my grandchildren; my mother and father; and my brothers, Jack, Allen, and Arnold.

PREFACE

I'm Stanley Rosenberg, an American-born body therapist living in Denmark. This book proposes a new approach to healing based on my experiences as a body therapist working within the framework of a completely new understanding of the function of the autonomic nervous system—the Polyvagal Theory, developed by Dr. Stephen Porges.

The autonomic nervous system not only regulates the workings of our visceral organs (stomach, lungs, heart, liver, etc.) but is closely tied to our emotional state, which directly influences our behavior. Thus the proper working of our autonomic nervous system is central to our emotional as well as physical health and well-being. Dr. Porges's Polyvagal framework has allowed me to achieve positive results with health issues as far-ranging as chronic obstructive pulmonary disease (COPD), migraine headaches, and autism—to name just a few.

I have been doing various forms of body therapy for more than forty-five years. That career was a far cry from Swarthmore College, from which I graduated in 1962 after majoring in English literature, philosophy, and history, participating in an intensive honors program. When I go to college reunions, I find that most of my friends became college professors, doctors, lawyers, psychologists, and other professionals. I am the only body therapist out of the two hundred and fifty students from my class.

BEHIND THE SCENES: THE PHILOSOPHY OF ACTING

During my time at Swarthmore I became interested in theater, and Japanese theater in particular. That led me to a graduate program in theater at the University of Hawaii, where we put on plays from Japan, China, India, and Thailand. After two years, I left the sandy beaches of Honolulu and moved to the crowded, dirty, noisy streets of the Lower East Side of Manhattan along with other young theater hopefuls.

From time to time, I helped Ellen Stewart, the producer of La MaMa, a popular off-off-Broadway theater where aspiring actors and directors put on new plays by hopeful but as yet undiscovered playwrights. I do not know whether it was my fate, my good luck, or my nose for finding good people to work with, but I was blessed that Ellen took me under her wing. After touring with her and a small theater troupe through Europe, Ellen insisted that I visit the Odin Theater, a small experimental venue in Denmark.

On Ellen's recommendation, I ended up as assistant to Eugenio Barba, director of the Odin Theater. Barba wanted the actors to create something new in every detail of their performance. On one occasion, Barba and his actors spent two days rehearsing one small scene—trying variations of staging, expressive body movements, and unusual patterns of vocal expression—that took only ninety seconds when it was finally finished and incorporated into the play.

Barba had been trained for three years as an assistant director at a Polish theater directed by Jerzy Grotowski, who had a reputation for doing some of the most exciting theater performances in the world at that time. Grotowski was both an innovative theater director and a theorist of the connections between mental, physical, and emotional processes. Grotowski's actors explored the physical and emotional aspects of extreme moments in the lives of their characters. They went into a world that was halfway between reality and fantasy, exploring dreamlike states invoked by traumatic experiences.

After three years as Grotowski's assistant. Barba also spent a year in India studying classical Kathakali dance theater, which uses extraordinary forms of stylized expression including masks, costumes, makeup, and frequent use of mime. To attain the high degree of flexibility and muscle control required for this art's body movements and footwork, Kathakali dancers undergo a strenuous course of training. To help them meet these challenges and achieve the necessary flexibility, they receive sessions of body massage.

All of these experiences influenced Barba and the Odin Theater; the acting training that I experienced there had its origins in Grotowski's work, and included acrobatics, yoga, and freestyle movement improvisation. I stayed at Barba's theater for an entire year, taking part in the daily training in voice, movement, and emotional expression.

In his "Statement of Principles," Grotowski wrote, "The main point then is that an actor should not try to acquire any kind of recipe or build up a "box of tricks." This is no place for collecting all sorts of means of expression."[1] My exposure to this philosophy at the Odin Theater shaped my approach to everything I did for the rest of my life, including learning and exploring body therapy.

In voice training, for example, we did not sing a song with a melody and text written by someone else. We did not try to imitate anything that we heard someone else do, but to explore the world of sounds that we generated in our own imagination—sounds that we had never heard anyone make before. This could take hours, days, or sometimes a week or more before I felt I had succeeded in making the exact sound I had imagined—and there was no one else who could judge whether I had made the "right" sound or not. Once I had made that sound, I never repeated it. I went on to the next sound that appeared in my imagination, and worked toward expressing that.

This same approach has manifested itself in my approach to bodywork. Alain Gehin, my primary teacher and mentor in craniosacral therapy, visceral massage, and osteopathic techniques, once said something very similar to what I'd learned at Odin Theater: "You learn techniques to understand principles. When you understand the principles, you will create your own techniques." He also continually emphasized one principle: "Test, treat, and then test again."

TAI CHI

Body therapy came naturally into my work of teaching actors. As a teacher and director, I pushed actors out of their comfort zones and beyond the usual limitations of their movement and vocal expression. We worked, for example, with mime and acrobatics. Along the way I found a short book on shiatsu massage, and I included that as part of our training to help the body move better.

While I was exploring the world of experimental theater in New York City, I also learned tai chi from Ed Young, a student and translator of

Professor Cheng Man-Ch'ing, one of the great tai chi masters of the twentieth century. Tai chi is unparalleled as a source of knowledge about natural ways of moving the body. Practicing the tai chi form every day is the kung fu of knowing yourself, similar to deeper forms of meditation in other traditions.

The movements of tai chi are continuous, spiraling, and "soft" compared with those of "hard" styles of self-defense such as karate, where the movements are in straight lines, fast, and with definite beginning and ending points. The goal of tai chi as a martial art is not to become stronger and faster than your opponent but to use your own body awareness, flexibility, and kinesthetic sense to find where your opponents are tense—and then "help" the opponents use their own force against themselves.

The ideal of tai chi is to use "a force of four ounces to deflect a thousand pounds." This concept has become an integral part of my body therapy. Some people doing massage and body therapies push hard into their client's body, with the intention of going deep. By contrast, I try to find the exact center of tension and the exact angle for me to push to increase the tension, and then use the minimum amount of force necessary to get the body to release itself. I often use no more than a few grams of pressure.

ROLFING AND OTHER INSIGHTS

After five years in New York, I moved back to Denmark and taught acting at the National Theater School for a year. Being a foreigner and trying to make headway in the Danish theater world without any network was harder than I had thought. So I decided to leave my work in theater and to support myself teaching tai chi and giving body therapy sessions.

In Denmark I kept hearing about Rolfing®, a form of hands-on body therapy created by Ida Rolf[2] that had the reputation at that time of being the gold standard of body therapy. (Rolfing is a form of "structural integration," the generic name for a form of connective-tissue massage that has the goal of helping clients have better posture, breathing, and movement.)

The idea of working from an inner intention, as we had done in our voice training at Odin Theater, came up in my discussions with Siegfried Libich, a German Rolfer. When he mentioned "working with intention" as an important element of Ida Rolf's teaching, I decided to take a series of ten Rolfing sessions with him. The effect of those sessions on me was so profound that I decided to learn the approach myself. I became one of the first of three Rolfers in Denmark, and I have now been working with this form of bodywork for more than thirty years.

In theater, actors usually take on the physical tensions of their characters, but in Rolfing we work to release the typical physical characteristics and habitual emotional patterns that limit our clients, restrict their movements, and cause pain and discomfort. The focus is on balancing tensions in the connective tissues of the body rather than "relaxing" the muscles, which is the usual approach to body therapy. The result is that they can move in new ways and have greater emotional flexibility. They can liberate themselves from clichés that have previously limited their freedom of expression, and move toward a more creative and authentic version of themselves.

Rolfers not only work with their hands; they also learn to read the body. Movement and postural analysis are an important part of the training that other modalities of body therapy had not yet begun to teach. Rolfers ask, "Where is the body out of balance? Where is the flow broken in a movement? What needs to be done to bring it back into shape?"

After I had been Rolfing for a few years, I began to hear other Rolfers talking about craniosacral therapy as a new frontier in body therapy. I went on to study that too, as well as other forms of osteopathic techniques including visceral massage and joint manipulation. During the following twenty-five-year period, I kept on learning from the best teachers I could find, attending advanced classes and trainings at least thirty days a year.

In Denmark I was able to develop my skills as a body therapist slowly, over more than four and a half decades. I am currently in my mid-seventies, and I believe that my life has moved more slowly here in Denmark than if I had followed a similar path doing body therapy in the United States, where financial opportunities are greater and more tempting, so that many successful therapists outgrow their practices and move on to other more lucrative endeavors. Also, I believe that the fashions regarding, which therapy is "in" and which is "out" change more quickly in the United States than in Denmark. I have been blessed to be able to follow my own path at my own tempo. Alain Gehin, my craniosacral teacher, said that becoming a skilled body therapist is not so much "knowing about" something intellectually but "learning how to do something with your hands." He claimed that a body therapist first begins to attain what the French call *savoir faire*—"know-how"—after giving ten thousand sessions. I have an image of myself, despite my American roots, as having apprenticed to become an Old-World European craftsman. I have had time to study, to practice, and to develop skills. I have had the luxury to be able to keep reaching for a greater level of finesse, sensitivity, and creativity with my hands.

All these ingredients were in the mixing bowl when I met Stephen Porges and was blown away by his new interpretation of how the autonomic nervous system functions—which I will explain later in this book.

INTRODUCTION:
THE AUTONOMIC NERVOUS SYSTEM

A discovery is said to be an accident meeting a prepared mind.

> —Albert Szent-Györgyi, Hungarian-born biochemist
> (1893–1986) who won the Nobel Prize for his discovery
> of Vitamin C in 1937[3]

*It doesn't matter how much you drive around, you will never
get to where you want to go if you don't have the right map.*

> —Stanley Rosenberg

I practiced various forms of body-oriented therapies for more than thirty years, but I eventually realized that I was using the wrong map. When I learned about Stephen Porges's Polyvagal Theory, his ideas expanded my understanding of how the autonomic nervous system functions, and immediately I had a better map.

The autonomic nervous system is an integral part of the human nervous system, monitoring and regulating the activity of the visceral organs—heart, lungs, liver, gall bladder, stomach, intestines, kidneys, and sexual organs. Problems with any of these organs can arise from dysfunction of the autonomic nervous system.

Before the Polyvagal Theory, there was a widely accepted belief that the autonomic nervous system functioned in two states: stress and relaxation. The stress response is a survival mechanism activated when we feel threatened; it mobilizes our body to prepare to fight or flee.[4] So in the stress state, our muscles are tense, thus enabling us to move faster and/or exert more power. The visceral organs work to support this extraordinary effort by our muscular system.

When we have won the fight and neutralized the threat, or when we have gotten far enough away so that we are no longer in danger, our relaxation response kicks in. We remain in this relaxed state until the next threat appears. In the old view of the autonomic nervous system, relaxation was characterized as the "rest and digest" or "feed and breed" state. This state was attributed to the activity of the vagus nerve, also known as the tenth cranial nerve, which, like all cranial nerves, originates in the brain or the brainstem. In this old, universally accepted interpretation, our autonomic nervous system vacillated between states of stress and relaxation.

However, problems arise when we get stuck in a stress state even when the threat or danger has passed, perhaps because our work or lifestyle is continually stressful. For many decades, chronic stress has been recognized as a health problem, with an enormous amount of scientific research devoted to understanding the harmful effects of long-term stress.

Attempts to treat and manage chronic stress spawned a widespread movement on the part of health-care practitioners, who wrote (and continue to write) a vast number of popular articles for a general audience in newspapers, magazines, books, and blogs. The pharmaceutical industry also began to provide a wide range of anti-stress drugs that have netted the corporations handsome profits as the use of these medications has soared. Yet, in spite of all these resources, many people continue to feel that they have not been helped sufficiently. They still feel stressed. Many believe that our society is getting more and more stressful every year, and that individuals are more stressed out as a result.

Perhaps the problem is that we have been using the wrong map. With the old understanding of the autonomic nervous system, we have not yet been able to find truly effective methods of stress management.

Like almost everyone working in the medical world and the alternative-therapy scene, I shared existing beliefs about the way that I thought the autonomic nervous system worked. Every day in my clinical practice, I used what I had learned about the old stress/relaxation model of the autonomic nervous system. The fact that my treatments worked served as a confirmation that this understanding of the autonomic nervous system was correct.

I enjoyed passing on what I had learned to students who wanted to acquire the various skills of body therapy that I had been using successfully. I taught the old model of autonomic nervous system function in all my courses in body therapy. As my classes filled, I founded a school, the Stanley Rosenberg Institute in Silkeborg, Denmark. In 1993 I invited a few of the therapists I had trained to teach some of the introductory courses so that I could concentrate on teaching the more advanced courses. Eventually other teachers took over the more advanced courses as well.

The specialty of our school was craniosacral therapy, which has its origins in the work of William Garner Sutherland (1873–1954), an American osteopath and the founder of osteopathy in the cranial field (OCF). (Osteopaths in the United States are licensed, with the same basic training and privileges as medical doctors.) While exploring dried cranial bones in an anatomy dissection lab, Sutherland found that he could fit the sawtooth edges of adjacent cranial bones together—but he noticed the possibility of slight movement between two adjacent bones. At the time, the belief was that if something existed in nature, there must be a reason for it. Sutherland postulated that the movement of the bones facilitated circulation of the cerebrospinal fluid, and he gathered techniques into what has become "craniosacral therapy."

CRANIAL BONE MOVEMENT

The cranial bones are held together by a system of elastic membranes that allow for slight movement between the individual bones. When Sutherland carefully palpated the bones of his patients' skulls, he was able to sense a slight but perceptible movement of the individual bones of the cranium in relationship to each other.

Sutherland noticed that many of his patients with medical problems originating in their nervous systems had restricted movement between the bones of their cranium. By releasing some of those tensions, he felt that the subtle movement of the bones was increased. This approach enabled him to help several of his patients with a wide variety of health issues that had not been helped by the usual medical treatments of medicine or surgery.

Whereas medical doctors tend to prescribe medicines to treat stress and other medical conditions, the craniosacral approach is a hands-on therapy that has proven to be particularly effective in improving the function of the nervous system. It can reduce chronic stress, release tensions in the muscular system, and bring better balance to the hormonal (endocrine) system. Sutherland developed therapeutic techniques in three areas: 1) releasing tension in the membranes; 2) releasing restrictions between the individual cranial bones; and 3) improving the flow of the cerebrospinal fluid.

THE BRAIN-BODY BARRIER

There is a physical structure made up of epithelial cells that envelop the brain and spinal cord. These cells form what is called the blood-brain barrier.

There is no direct circulation of blood directly to the neurons of the brain and spinal cord. Instead, the tissues of these structures are surrounded by colorless cerebrospinal fluid, which circulates to deliver necessary nourishment to the cells of the brain and spinal cord and to carry away waste products of cellular metabolism before returning to the blood.

The cerebrospinal fluid is found in small amounts in the blood throughout the entire body, but it is finer than the rest of the blood. It contains no red or white blood cells, and fewer impurities than blood.

In the brain the cerebrospinal fluid is filtered out of the blood and circulates through the cranium in the spaces surrounding the brain and spinal cord. After circulating around the brain and spinal cord, the cerebrospinal fluid returns to the jugular veins, where it rejoins the blood returning to the heart from the rest of the body. Then it is circulated from the heart and freshened by the lungs and kidneys.

The blood supply to the brainstem and the nerves arising there is crucial to the function of the five cranial nerves whose function is necessary for the state of social engagement, which includes the ventral branch of the vagus nerve.

Removing restrictions to this blood supply is at the core of successfully improving the function of the ventral branch of the vagus nerve and the other four cranial nerves necessary to social engagement. Some of the best ways to achieve this are found in the domain of craniosacral osteopathy.

For decades, craniosacral education was the exclusive domain of osteopathic physicians. They traditionally restricted attendance in their courses to licensed osteopaths and students enrolled in osteopathic medical schools. However, some of the hands-on disciplines were eventually taught to non-osteopathic physicians and students. Because many of those techniques were so effective, an eager market for them developed among practitioners of alternative and complementary therapies.

One American osteopath, John Upledger, broke with tradition and began teaching craniosacral techniques to non-osteopaths. Much of the focus of Upledger's work was on unwinding the tension in the membranes. He founded the Upledger Institute, where I took my first course in craniosacral therapy in 1983. Craniosacral therapy has now become popular with alternative therapists all over the world.

In 1995, after I had been successfully practicing what I had learned from the Upledger Institute, I went on to study with Alain Gehin, a French osteopath who specialized in biomechanical craniosacral therapy. His focus was on releasing tension in the connective tissue spanning adjacent cranial bones, thereby allowing them to move more freely.[5]

A few years after that I took introductory courses in biomechanical craniosacral therapy, which focuses on increasing the circulation of the cerebrospinal fluid. All three approaches have the same goal that Sutherland espoused—to improve the function of the craniosacral system.

MY OWN CLINICAL PRACTICE

In my own practice I preferred biomechanical craniosacral therapy, which reminded me of my work with Rolfing. BCT is specific; it helped me find the exact places in the cranial joints that needed releasing and provided me with more than 150 specific techniques to release these tensions. This powerful approach often effectively restores the function of the cranial nerves in a short period of time.

In my clinic, in addition to treating clients with craniosacral therapy, I gave individual sessions in Rolfing, which balances the myofascia (*myo-* means "muscle"; *fascia* refers to connective tissue). I also offered sessions in visceral massage to improve the function of the digestive and respiratory systems. As I worked with techniques from these various modalities, I observed changes in the client's nervous system in terms of stress and relaxation during the course of a hands-on treatment.

My work with patients was extremely successful. As time went on, more and more people wanted to learn my techniques, and the Stanley Rosenberg Institute grew to employ twelve teachers working on a part-time basis. Courses were taught in Danish. In Denmark alone we educated several hundred students over several years. These therapists in turn treated thousands of patients. My reputation spread beyond the borders of Denmark, and I taught in several other countries as well.

The idea of the two-state (stress and relaxation) function of the autonomic nervous system played a prominent role in our curriculum. I taught about it in my classes on craniosacral therapy, visceral massage, and connective-tissue release. Together with an American neurologist, Ronald Lawrence, MD, I even wrote a book, *Pain Relief with Osteomassage,*[6] about pain relief and hands-on treatment, based on this interpretation of the autonomic nervous system.

When I first heard Stephen Porges lecture about his Polyvagal Theory in Baltimore in 2001, I had been working successfully with body-oriented therapies for almost thirty-five years. Porges's theory, however, was right up my alley, and it gave me a whole new outlook on the autonomic nervous system. This in turn gave me a new and more effective way to help my patients.

Porges's Polyvagal Theory brought about a revolutionary advancement in my understanding of the autonomic nervous system. According to this theory, five cranial nerves (CNs) must function adequately in order to attain the desirable state of social engagement. These five nerves are CN V, VII, IX, X, and XI, and they all originate in the brainstem.

Before I heard Porges speak, I had studied anatomy with Professor Patrick Coughlin, who taught us about each of the twelve cranial nerves, including the vagus nerve (CN X), and how to test their function. I had also learned specific biomechanical hands-on techniques from my craniosacral teacher Alain Gehin to improve the function of the twelve cranial nerves. So I was well prepared for an infusion of insight offered by the Polyvagal Theory. I adapted the techniques I had learned to successfully address a wide range of maladies with this new paradigm.

I believe that the information and exercises in this book can be usefully implemented by almost anyone, from beginner to experienced craniosacral therapist, to improve cranial-nerve function in themselves and their patients, and to obtain relief from many unpleasant symptoms, conditions, and health issues—especially those that have been difficult to diagnose and heal.

THE NEUROLOGY OF SOCIAL ENGAGEMENT

Spinal nerves originate in the brain, make up part of the spinal cord, exit the spinal cord between adjacent vertebrae, and then go to various areas throughout the body. A spinal nerve is a mixed nerve, carrying motor, sensory, and autonomic signals between the spinal cord and corresponding regions of the body.

Some of the fibers of the spinal nerves weave together to make up the sympathetic chain, which runs the length of the spine from vertebrae T1 to L2. (T1 is the first thoracic vertebrae and L2 is the second lumbar vertebra). This chain supports the activity of the visceral organs and muscles when a person is mobilized by a threat of danger into a "fight or flight" response.

Cranial nerves, except for cranial nerves I (olfactory) and II (optic), originate in the brainstem, at the base of the brain. (See the illustrations "Brain" and "Cranial Nerves" in the Appendix.) They then make their way to various structures in both the cranium and the rest of the body. Some cranial nerves, for instance, innervate the muscles of facial expression, while others go to the heart, lungs, stomach, and other organs of digestion. Some cranial nerves go to the muscles that move the eyes, while others connect to cells in the nose to enable our sense of smell.

According to the Polyvagal Theory, when a person is feeling safe—not threatened or in danger—and if her body is healthy and functioning well, she can enjoy a physiological state that supports spontaneous social engagement behaviors. Social engagement, neurologically speaking, is a state based on the activity of five cranial nerves: the ventral branch of the vagus nerve (cranial nerve X), and pathways within cranial nerves V, VII, IX, and XI.

When working together properly, the activity of these five nerves supports a state that enables social interaction, communication, and appropriate self-soothing behaviors. When we are socially engaged, we can experience feelings of love and friendship. And when individual members of a group can come together and cooperate with others, it enhances everyone's chances for survival.

Other inherent values derive from social engagement: we bond with each other, develop friendships, and enjoy intimate sexual relationships; we communicate, talk with each other, care for each other, work together, raise families, tell stories, play sports, sing together, dance together, and entertain one another. We enjoy sitting at a table and sharing a meal or a drink with friends and loved ones. Social engagement might arise when a parent puts a child to sleep, lying close and reading a book or telling a story until the child drifts off, or in the intimate moment experienced by two lovers lying close to each other after they have made love. These are some of the important experiences that make us human beings.

Social interaction is not reserved for our relations with other people. We love our pets, we feed them, and we go for walks with our dogs. We often talk to our pets, and we are quite sure that they understand what we are saying. When they reciprocate with signs of affection, we feel happy. Almost anyone recognizes these activities, experiences, and qualities arising from the state of social engagement. However, these kinds of activities and interactions are neither described nor explained by the old model of the autonomic nervous system.

Being together with others in positive ways is not only facilitated by the social engagement circuit of the autonomic nervous system; positive experiences with others also help us to regulate our autonomic nervous system. When we are together with other people who are socially engaged, we feel better. On the other hand, when we do not have enough positive social interactions with others, we can easily become stressed, depressed, asocial, or even antisocial.

This new understanding of the multifaceted roles of the cranial nerves, and particularly their connection with the state of social engagement, enabled me to consistently help more people with an even wider range of health issues. All I had to do was to determine whether these five cranial nerves functioned well and, if not, to use a technique to get them to function better.

This made it possible for me to achieve far greater success in my practice and to treat intransigent conditions such as migraine headaches, depression, fibromyalgia, COPD, post-traumatic stress, forward head posture, and neck and shoulder problems, among others.

This book is an introduction to the theory and practice of Polyvagal healing. After describing basic neurological structures, I will list some of the physical, psychological, and social issues caused by dysfunctions of those five cranial nerves.

According to the Polyvagal Theory, the autonomic nervous system has two other functions in addition to those of the ventral branch of the vagus nerve: the activity of the dorsal branch of the vagus nerve, and sympathetic activity from the spinal chain. This multiple *(poly-)* nature of the vagus nerve gives the theory its name.

The differences between the functions of the ventral and dorsal branches of the vagus nerve have profound implications for physical and behavioral health and healing. Throughout the book, I propose a new approach to healing that includes self-help exercises and hands-on therapeutic techniques that are simple to learn and easy to use. It is my hope that this knowledge will continue to spread and enable many more people to help themselves and others.

RESTORING SOCIAL ENGAGEMENT

I have written this book to make the benefits of restoring vagal function available to a broad range of people, even if they have no prior experience with craniosacral or other forms of hands-on therapy. Readers can acquire a unique set of easy-to-learn and easy-to-do self-help exercises and hands-on techniques that should enable them to improve the function of these five nerves in themselves and others. I used the principles behind Alain Gehin's work to develop these techniques.

The exercises and techniques restore flexibility to the functioning of the autonomic nervous system. They can help eliminate the general adverse conditions of chronic stress, which arises from the overstimulation of the spinal sympathetic chain, and depressive behavior and shutdown, which arise from activity in the dorsal vagal circuit. The exercises are noninvasive and do not involve medicine or surgery. The improvements in ventral vagus nerve function from doing the exercises help to regulate the visceral organs involved in breathing, digestion, elimination, and sexual function.

I tested the exercises with more than a hundred patients in my clinic before introducing the techniques to closely monitored groups in my classes and lectures. My conclusion was that my new approach using the exercises in this book will enhance most people's health and their capability for social engagement. The positive effects may last for a surprisingly long time.

However, life is challenging, and nothing is permanent. While our goal is to help make the autonomic nervous system resilient, social engagement is not a permanent condition. Nor can we always prevent a person from encountering threatening circumstances or dangerous situations.

The body, the nervous system, and the emotions continually adapt to help us respond to changing conditions. If we are threatened, or in physical or emotional danger, it is appropriate for our autonomic nervous system to respond physiologically with a temporary state of sympathetic activity in the spinal chain, or with dorsal vagal activity. These changes help us to survive. Once the actual threat or danger is over, it is best if we can bounce back into a state of social engagement.

Because nothing in the body lasts forever, though, the nervous system may slide back from social engagement into a state of activity of the spinal sympathetic chain or the dorsal vagal circuit. In this case, repeating the exercises should quickly restore ventral vagal function and leave the person in a socially engaged state again. It may be necessary to repeat these exercises or techniques occasionally or regularly.

The positive effects are cumulative. Our autonomic nervous system becomes more resilient each time we can restore a state of social engagement following activation of the spinal sympathetic chain or the dorsal vagus branch. We can do so by using the Basic Exercise, a very simple self-help technique described in Part Two. Our long-term goal is to encourage the autonomic nervous system to return naturally, on its own, from a state of stress (spinal sympathetic activation) or depression (activity in the dorsal vagal circuit) to a state of social engagement, as soon as conditions change for the better and we return to feeling physically and emotionally safe.

The techniques and exercises in Part Two help to improve movement of the head, neck, and shoulders, and to correct some of the postural and functional issues that we attribute to aging: forward head posture, kyphosis, dowager's hump, flat lower back, reduced breathing capacity, etc. Every time that you utilize the techniques in this book, you will notice improvement.

PART ONE

ANATOMICAL FACTS OLD AND NEW: THE POLYVAGAL THEORY

Overcoming Health Challenges: Are You Fighting the Heads of the Hydra?

Many people struggle with health issues. Often their stories are reminiscent of the contest portrayed in Greek mythology between Hercules, the strongest of all men, and the water beast named Hydra. Hercules was half god and half human; his father was Zeus, god of the sky and thunder, who ruled all the other gods on Olympus. Greatest of all heroes, Hercules was sent on a mission to kill Hydra, a snake-like water beast with many heads.

Hercules had a golden sword that had been given to him by Athena. In Greek mythology, Athena—the patron of the city-state of Athens—was the goddess of wisdom, civilization, just warfare, strength, strategy, female arts, crafts, justice, and skill, who often accompanied heroes in their battles.

Hydra was a dangerous opponent—even her breath was poisonous. For each of Hydra's many heads that Hercules cut off with his sword, the seemingly immortal Hydra grew two new heads. Realizing that he could not defeat Hydra by cutting off her heads one at a time, Hercules summoned his nephew Iolaus for help. Iolaus came up with the idea of using a blazing firebrand to scorch the neck stumps after each decapitation, making it impossible for two heads to grow back in the same place.

Luckily for Hercules, Hydra had one weak spot: one of her heads was mortal. When Hercules found Hydra's mortal head and cut it off, Hydra finally died.

The mythical Hydra is a metaphor for the frustration of treating one symptom only to have one or more others crop up in its place. Like the multiple heads of Hydra, multiple health issues plague many of us, and chasing symptoms one at a time with a medicine or an operation for each may give temporary relief but does not necessarily root out the source.

We might take a pill for one health problem, another pill for another problem, and a third to counteract the side effects of the first two pills. We may even take multiple different pills every day. But often the pills only help temporarily, if at all, and sometimes we have to continue to take them for the rest of our lives.

Our society primarily relies on two approaches in conventional medicine: biochemical (drugs) and surgical. These powerful tools are valuable in some cases and have helped many people, including myself. Surgical operations can be life saving. But even the best of operations leave scar tissue, which can restrict movement by making it more difficult for layers of muscles and connective tissue to slide freely on adjacent layers.

Also, there are many symptoms, conditions, and health issues that are not debilitating or life threatening; often, lacking viable alternatives, we try to treat these issues with the usual medical approach of prescription drugs and/or surgery. These may not be the best solutions, however. In many cases they do not work as effectively as we wish, and often they produce undesirable side effects.

Like fighting the Hydra, our symptom-suppression often just results in more symptoms popping up. For achieving lasting health, by contrast, there is a largely untapped potential in understanding how the nervous system works and approaching difficult health issues in a new way. Simply stated: if the ventral branch of the vagus nerve is not functioning, make it functional. Since the autonomic nervous system regulates important functions of the body such as circulation, respiration, digestion, and reproduction, a wide range of consequences can ensue if the vagus and other cranial nerves are not working properly.

Below is a partial list of common problems that can arise from the autonomic nervous system. These are symptoms that affect many people. Have you experienced any of these symptoms or know people who suffer from them? If so, read on, because working with the cranial nerves can bring relief.

The Heads of the Hydra:
Common Problems Related to Cranial-Nerve Dysfunction

Chronic physical tensions

- Tense/hard muscles
- Sore neck and shoulder muscles
- Migraines
- Back pain
- Tightly clenched teeth
- Grinding teeth at night
- Eye or facial tensions
- Cold hands and feet
- Unwarranted sweating
- Tenseness after exertion
- Arthritis
- Nervousness
- Dizziness
- Lump in the throat

Emotional issues

- Irritability, anger
- Feeling "down"
- Feeling of hopelessness
- Lack of energy
- Tendency to cry easily
- General anxiety
- Feeling of heaviness
- Extended periods of depression
- Fearfulness
- Nightmares

- Restlessness
- Difficulty sleeping
- Excessive worries
- Difficulty concentrating
- Forgetfulness
- Frustration
- Excessive daydreaming and fantasizing

Heart and lung problems

- Chest pains
- Asthma
- Hyperventilation
- Shortness of breath
- Irregular heartbeat
- High blood pressure

Visceral-organ dysfunctions

- Poor digestion
- Constipation
- Irritation of the large intestine
- Diarrhea
- Stomach problems
- Hyperacidity, ulcer, heartburn
- Loss of appetite
- Excessive eating

Immune-system problems

- Frequent influenza
- Minor infections
- Allergies

Behavioral problems

- Frequent accidents or injuries
- Increase in drinking or smoking

- Excessive use of medicine with or without prescription
- Autism, ADHD, Asperger's syndrome

Interpersonal relationships

- Excessive or unreasonable distrust
- Difficulty in reaching agreements
- Loss of interest in sex

Mental issues

- Excessive worrying
- Difficulty concentrating
- Difficulty remembering
- Difficulty making decisions

Other problems

- Excessive menstrual pains
- Skin problems

Given the challenges and stresses that we face in our lives, everyone is troubled by one or more of these symptoms from time to time. At first glance, this list seems to include unrelated problems—we could classify some of them as "physical," some as "mental," others as "emotional," and still others as "behavioral." Making such distinctions by grouping symptoms is not helpful in this context, however, and distracts from the observation that the underlying physiological cause is essentially the same.

Usually people have more than one of these symptoms at the same time. The scientific term for this is *comorbidity.* The symptoms can disappear and recur at irregular intervals. If the symptoms occur rarely and are not debilitating, they are not so much of a problem. However, if the problems occur often, or most of the time, it is advisable to address them.

Rather than treating individual symptoms as separate issues with a pill to be taken for each one, it would be preferable to find a common thread that links them. Perhaps we can we find a simple, effective treatment that can mitigate or terminate these many seemingly separate issues—perhaps we can find the Hydra's mortal head.

The common thread may be a fairly simple one: All of the problems in this list occur at least partly from dorsal vagal activity or activation of the spinal sympathetic nervous system, and can be addressed by reinstating normal function of the ventral vagus nerve branch and other nerves required for social engagement.

The idea that cranial nerves play a role in any of these health issues is almost universally overlooked by contemporary medicine. Most people do not know much about the brainstem, where these nerves originate, nor about the cranial nerves themselves.

I believe, and have repeatedly confirmed, that if we can get the five nerves that support social engagement to function properly, there is a good chance of alleviating or eliminating many of the symptoms on the list. This belief is based on my own clinical experience over several decades, and the experiences of the hundreds of therapists that I have trained at the Stanley Rosenberg Institute.

CHAPTER 1

Get to Know Your Autonomic Nervous System

The human nervous system has one primary function: to ensure the survival of our physical body. The nervous system is composed of the brain, the brainstem, the cranial nerves, the spinal cord, the spinal nerves, and the enteric nerves. The focus of our attention here is the autonomic nervous system, which is made up of elements of the brainstem, some of the cranial nerves, and some parts of some of the spinal nerves.

The Twelve Cranial Nerves

Writing about the function of the twelve cranial nerves for a range of readers with extensive to zero knowledge about them has been a challenge. How can I introduce the subject to readers hearing about these nerves for the first time, while also helping knowledgeable people to understand cranial nerve function in a new and useful way?

For readers new to the subject, I will present a simple description of the function of each of the twelve cranial nerves. If you are already familiar with the cranial nerves, I hope to present a new perspective and some new information about their function.

Cranial nerves are different from spinal nerves. Some cranial nerves connect the brainstem with organs and muscles of the head such as the nose, eyes, ears, and tongue. The brainstem extends from the brain; it lies on the underside of the brain and is the beginning of the spinal cord. (See "Brain," "Cranial nerves," and "Spinal cord" in the Appendix.) Other cranial nerves go through small openings in the cranium to reach the throat, face, neck, thorax, and abdomen. Each of the twelve cranial nerves has pathways on both the right and left sides.

One of the cranial nerves "wanders" through the body, coursing from the brainstem into the chest and abdomen to regulate many of the visceral organs. It innervates the muscles of the throat (pharynx and larynx), and the organs of respiration (lungs), circulation (heart), digestion (stomach, liver, pancreas, duodenum, small intestine, and the ascending and transverse sections of the large intestine), and elimination (kidneys). Because this nerve is so long and has so many branches, it was named the "vagus" nerve, from the Latin word *vagus,* meaning "vagrant, wanderer."

The vagus nerve helps to regulate a vast array of bodily functions necessary for maintaining homeostasis. Whereas the sympathetic chain extends from the spinal nerves and supports the state of stress and mobilization for survival, several of the cranial nerves support non-stress states. One of the primary functions of the cranial nerves is to facilitate rest and restitution. They also enable the senses of sight, smell, taste, and hearing, as well as the sense of touch on the skin of the face. In mammals, some of the cranial nerves work together to facilitate and promote social behavior.

Each cranial nerve is numbered with a Roman numeral; for example, the olfactory nerve is also called CN I, meaning "first cranial nerve." Note that although the nerves are paired, the singular term is usually used, so that "CN I" actually refers to a pair of nerves.

The cranial nerves are numbered based on their location. They extend from a half-circle on each side of the brain; an early anatomist assigned the number CN I to the topmost nerve, CN II to the next nerve down in the half-circle, and so on.

THE VARIOUS FUNCTIONS OF CRANIAL NERVES

As the fibers within a conduit often have different functions, a cranial nerve may have multiple functions as well. When we first look at the various cranial nerves, their functions seem to be unrelated. For example, one of the nerves helps us swallow, another tightens a muscle that rotates the eyeball toward the midline, and a third helps to regulate blood pressure.

However, though it is not usually noted in the study of anatomy, all twelve cranial nerves have one thing in common: they are all involved in helping us to find food; chew, swallow, and digest; and eliminate undigested food as waste.

Cranial nerves control the secretion of enzymes and acids in the mouth and stomach, the production of bile in the liver and storage of bile in the gall bladder, and the production and storage of digestive enzymes in the pancreas. They monitor and regulate the movement of undigested food all the way from the stomach to the transverse colon. They control the release of gall and pancreatic enzymes into the duodenum, in appropriate amounts and at appropriate times, to digest the food and break down its composition. After the proteins, carbohydrates, and fats have been sufficiently broken down, these nutrients can be absorbed through the walls of the small intestine.

We will start this discussion of the individual cranial nerves by noting how each one contributes to the digestive process. Then we will look at some additional functions of the cranial nerves that are not related to food, such as regulation of the kidneys and bladder, the heart and respiration, and sex and reproduction.

If you have never heard of cranial nerves before, do not worry about remembering which nerves have which functions; you can always come back to this section and refresh your memory with the table on page 12. What will be most useful is to get a general impression of the kinds of functions regulated by these nerves, including the state of social engagement. If you have studied the twelve cranial nerves before, the following will present a somewhat different approach to help broaden your understanding.

The olfactory nerve, or CN I, enables our sense of smell. In terms of evolution, CN I was the first of the cranial nerves to develop. The sense of smell is vital to human beings and all other mammals; it is crucial in first finding food and then determining whether a morsel is edible. Smells create an immediate response of attraction or repulsion—does my mouth water when I bring the morsel closer, or do I turn my head away in disgust?

Our response to smells is powerful, primitive, and instinctual, so various smells have strong emotional impacts on us. It is important for a baby to recognize the smell of its mother, and for sexual partners to smell each other in order to intensify their arousal.

The nerve fibers of CN I originate in sensory organs in the nose and have a direct pathway to the forebrain. CN I is the only cranial nerve with direct transmission from the sensory organs to the brain without intermediary synapses. (A synapse is a structure that permits a neuron, or nerve cell, to pass an electrical or chemical signal to another cell, neural or otherwise.)

The olfactory nerve is thus the only cranial nerve that transmits information (smell) directly to the cerebral cortex without relaying it through another part of the central nervous system. Interestingly, this part of our "old brain" is instrumental in the formation of memory, which makes sense from the standpoint of survival. This is why smells make up some of our strongest and most evocative memories.

Other cranial nerves enable our vision, and sight of course plays a critical role in helping us to find food. CN II, the optic nerve, also originates in the forebrain. It transmits signals from the rods and cones in the retina of the eye to a synapse, and across that synapse to the visual centers in the back (occipital) lobe of the cerebral cortex. The brain interprets these nerve impulses into what we see.

We might be searching for something to eat, and see something interesting. Can we recognize it from past experience? Does it look like food? Does it look fresh? Is it free from mold and discoloration? If it looks good, we then might decide to bring it closer to our face so that we can smell it, and then we might put it into our mouth to taste it.

Moving our eyeballs in different directions expands our field of vision. The small muscles that move the eyeballs are controlled by three other cranial nerves: CN III (oculomotor), IV (trochlear), and VI (abducens). These allow us to roll our eyes up, down, right, or left.

We can extend our field of vision even further if we use the neck muscles to move our head. CN XI, the spinal accessory nerve, controls the trapezius and sternocleidomastoid muscles. These muscles move our head so that we can look up, down, and to the sides. This allows our search for food to include bringing a morsel closer to smell it and, if it does not smell good, to turn our head away.

However, sight and smell alone do not tell us for sure that something is edible. We take the next step and put it into our mouth: does it taste all right? In order to taste properly, we need to mix the food with saliva. The secretion of saliva is controlled by the CN V (trigeminal), CN VII (facial), and CN IX (glossopharyngeal) nerves that innervate the salivary glands. Saliva not only increases our ability to taste things, it also initiates the digestive process by beginning starch breakdown and moistening food, making it easier to swallow.

To mix the food with saliva, we use CN V (the trigeminal nerve) to innervate the muscles of mastication, opening and closing the jaw and grinding the food with a side-to-side movement. We use CN XII (the hypoglossal nerve) to move our tongue to shift the food around in the mouth, and on and off the surfaces of our teeth. We use CN VII (the facial nerve) to relax and tighten the muscles of the cheeks, creating a pouch for the food and emptying it to move food back onto the grinding surfaces of the teeth. We also help move the food around with the muscles of the lips, which are also innervated by CN VII.

For the actual tasting of food, we use the taste buds on the tongue, which connect to branches of three cranial nerves: CN VII (the facial nerve), CN IX (the glossopharyngeal nerve), and CN X (the vagus nerve). Does the food taste all right, or is there a strange taste signaling that the morsel might be dangerous to eat? If the food does not taste good, we can easily spit it out before we swallow it, and avoid becoming sick or poisoned.

If we decide to swallow, the tongue flips this chewed food mixed with saliva to the top of the esophagus, at the back of the mouth. The esophagus is a muscular tube that moves food from the throat to the stomach, contracting rhythmically in the same way that the intestines do. We swallow food with muscles in the throat that are innervated by CN IX, the glossopharyngeal nerve, and tongue muscles innervated by CN XII, the hypoglossal nerve, as well as other muscles innervated by CN V and CN VII.

The upper third of the esophagus is innervated by the ventral branch of the vagus nerve, while the rest of the esophagus is innervated by the dorsal vagus branch.

If we sense that something is wrong with the food once it reaches the stomach, the old (dorsal) vagus branch gives us one last chance to regurgitate it before it continues into the small intestine. Our gag reflex is controlled on both ends of the esophagus, by the glossopharyngeal nerve (CN IX) at the top and the vagus (CN X) lower down. It's easy to see how complicated the act of swallowing actually is, requiring the coordinated function of many cranial nerves!

The cranial nerves assist in the search for food in other ways. Many animals locate possible prey using their finely attuned sense of hearing. Most anatomical sources consider CN VIII, the auditory nerve,[7] to be the only cranial nerve that facilitates hearing. However, in mammals, the trigeminal (CN V) and facial (CN VII) nerves also have important roles to play in listening and in understanding human speech by regulating the middle-ear muscles. Tightening or relaxing tension levels in the eardrum, with the help of these nerves, changes the loudness of specific acoustic frequencies that pass through the eardrum to the inner ear. When the levels of sound are too strong for the fine mechanism of the inner ear, the stapedius muscle dampens the vibrations. (For more about hearing, see Chapter 7.)

Major Functions of the Cranial Nerves

CN I	Olfactory nerve	Smell; helps to locate food
CN II	Optic nerve	Vision; makes it possible to see
CN III	Oculomotor nerve	Looking; controls some eyeball muscles
CN IV	Trochlear nerve`	Looking; controls some eyeball muscles
CN V	Trigeminal nerve	Chewing and swallowing Hearing; *tensor tympani* muscle
CN VI	Abducens nerve	Looking; controls some eyeball muscles
CN VII	Facial nerve	Chewing; some facial muscles and salivary secretions Hearing; stapedius muscle
CN VIII	Acoustic nerve	Hearing; translates sound waves into nerve impulses
CN IX	Glossopharyngeal nerve	Swallowing

CN X	New vagus nerve	The new (ventral) vagus branch innervates
	Old vagus nerve	and controls the upper third of the esophagus and most of the pharyngeal muscles, and it regulates the heart and bronchi.
		The old (dorsal) vagus branch innervates the lower two-thirds of the esophagus; it regulates stomach function, digestive glands and organs such as liver and gall bladder, and movement of food through the intestines (except the descending colon).
CN XI	Spinal accessory nerve	Innervates the trapezius and sternocleidomastoid muscles, which turn the head and expand the visual field
CN XII	Hypoglossal nerve	Moves the tongue

In addition to eating, several other functions are performed by the cranial nerves. The visceral afferent (sensory) branches of cranial nerves V, VII, IX, X, and XI gather information from our visceral organs: Are we safe, threatened, or in mortal danger? Does our body feel healthy, or is there an imbalance, pain, dysfunction, or illness? If we are safe and healthy, these nerves facilitate the desirable state of social engagement.

Cranial Nerve Dysfunction and Social Engagement

We consider "normal" human behavior to be an expression of positive social values. Our actions should be beneficial for our own survival and well-being, as well as for the well-being of others.

When we are socially engaged, it is easy for other people to understand our behavior, and what we do makes sense to others; most of us are socially engaged most of the time. However, sometimes we temporarily drop into a state of chronic activation of the spinal sympathetic chain system (fight or flight) or of dorsal vagal activity (withdrawal, shutdown). Then, if our autonomic nervous system is resilient, we will soon bounce back up to a state of social engagement.

Unfortunately, some of us are not socially engaged most of the time; if we lack the necessary resilience to spontaneously come back to a state of social engagement, we become stuck in sympathetic-chain or dorsal vagal states. In these states it is often hard for other people to understand our values, motivation, and behavior. Our actions seem irrational, often run counter to our own best interests, and can be destructive to ourselves and others. If we are not socially engaged, it makes life difficult not only for ourselves but for those around us.

Let's take a look at the five cranial nerves necessary for social engagement, and what kinds of problems can arise when they are not functioning properly. These symptoms provide a clue that someone is not socially engaged; a person with these symptoms might benefit from treatment of the affected nerve(s).

THE FIFTH AND SEVENTH CRANIAL NERVES

CN V, the trigeminal nerve, has several motor functions including control of the muscles of mastication that move the jaw when we chew. CN V also has sensory functions, and it receives impulses from the sensory nerves of the skin of the face.

CN VII, the facial nerve, also has several motor functions. It controls the tensing and relaxing of the individual muscles of the face. Changes in the pattern of tensions in our facial muscles create our facial expressions, which not only communicate different emotions but also reflect our internal states in terms of health or illness. Ideally, changes in facial expressions are spontaneous and reflect the flow of changing emotions and thoughts.

Is someone's face deadpan, lacking animation? This is usually a sign of CN VII dysfunction. We can make faces voluntarily—for example, putting on a smile or opening our eyes wide. But these are not the same as spontaneous facial expressions.

Spontaneous small changes in facial expression (or lack thereof) in this transverse stripe from the corners of the eyes to the corners of the lips, whether consciously or unconsciously noticed by others, can reveal whether or not we are socially engaged.

In addition to these separate functions, CN V and CN VII have inter-related functions. CN VII innervates the muscles of the face, and CN V is a sensory nerve to the skin of the face. When we change facial expression, this gives us the "feel of the face." Both nerves play a role in listening to and understanding what is being said, enabling us to take part in a conversation. This is also crucial to facilitating social engagement.

The stapedius, the smallest muscle in the body, is innervated by CN VII. This muscle protects the inner ear from high noise levels, primarily the volume of your own voice. The roar of a lion can be deafening, striking terror in other animals to the point of paralyzing them. The lion protects itself from the sound of its own voice by tightening its own stapedius muscle an instant before it roars, so that it is not affected by the loud noise.

By reducing the volume of sounds above and below the frequency of the human female voice, the stapedius muscle allows a baby to more clearly hear her mother's voice. If you are easily disturbed by background noises, your stapedius muscle might not be doing its job of reducing the volume of the low-frequency sounds, making it hard for you to hear what someone else is saying in a noisy room.

Hyperacusis, another hearing problem, can result from dysfunction of the stapedius as well as another muscle in the middle ear, the *tensor tympani*, or eardrum muscle, innervated by CN V. As this muscle tightens, it increases the tension, which diminishes sound. This is a useful function when we eat, reducing the level of noise from chewing. (For more about hyperacusis and stapedius dysfunction, see Chapter 7.)

Dysfunctions of CN V and CN VII are quite common in adults, often coming as an undesirable side effect of tooth extractions or orthodontic braces. I have observed in several of my clients who have had dental work that the pterygoid process of their sphenoid bone and the palatine bone (one of the small facial bones) in their hard palate are "pulled out of joint" in relationship to each other. As part of my training in biomechanical craniosacral therapy, I learned to look at the shape of the hard palate to see whether the palatine bone has been displaced laterally, and to perform a technique to bring this bone back to its proper position.

Some of the branches of CN V and CN VII meet in this area. A very slight misalignment of the facial bones in the joint between the sphenoid and palatine bones can put pressure on both nerves. I sometimes treat clients who have had problems in these two nerves after having had a tooth pulled. When I ask dentists about pain in a tooth and misalignment of these two bones, most of them know exactly what I mean. They often respond that they are very careful not to pull a tooth just on the basis of pain if there is no sign of infection.

However, I also meet people whose dentist did not learn this, or perhaps forgot it. One woman had a pain in a tooth after an extraction of a different tooth. Her dentist pulled the second tooth, but this did not alleviate the pain. He did not seem to know that the nerves in this joint could be compressed from a displacement of these two bones in relationship to each other. This dentist was persistent in his attempt to help the woman to be free of pain; he pulled another tooth, and then another. When she came to me, she had almost no teeth left in her mouth—and still had the same pain.

I presently have another client who started to grind his teeth at night after a tooth was pulled out. Many dentists do not recognize the problem, or perhaps do not have the skills to address it.

In my first session, I generally ask all my clients if they have had a tooth extracted, or if they wore orthodontic braces. Either of these can cause chronic spinal sympathetic stimulation or a chronic dorsal vagal state.

The sphenoid bone is the most centrally located bone in the cranium. The outer surfaces of the sphenoid bone make up what we commonly call the temples. If a boxer takes a punch on one of the temples, he risks being knocked out cold. Many boxers know this, and target the temples of their opponent. If they hit the temple, they will almost surely win by knockout. It is also why baseball batters wear a cap with flaps that protect their temples from injury if they are hit by a ball. The innermost part of the sphenoid bone has a saddle-like depression in which the pituitary gland rests.

When one branch of a cranial nerve is under direct physical pressure, not only that branch but other branches of that nerve can become dysfunctional. Thus a dislocation between the sphenoid and palatine bones can result in dysfunction of the nerves to the face and middle ear; this is enough to block the entire social-engagement nervous system.

Cranial nerve V goes to the skin of the face, while cranial nerve VII goes to the muscles of the face. To correct some of these dysfunctions and to give yourself a natural "facelift," Part Two of this book includes a technique that stimulates both the fifth and seventh cranial nerves. Although you should notice an improvement in reducing facial tensions the very first time you do the exercise, it is a good idea to repeat it occasionally, especially if you have lost your natural smile because of being in a dorsal vagal or spinal-sympathetic state.

Two other muscles innervated by CN V are the medial and lateral pterygoids, which arise on the sphenoid bone and help to open and close the jaw. A slight displacement of this bone can cause irregularities such as overbite, underbite, or crossbite.

THE NINTH, TENTH, AND ELEVENTH CRANIAL NERVES

One of the two branches of the tenth cranial nerve (the ventral vagus) arises in a structure called the *nucleus ambiguus* in the brainstem, along with the ninth and eleventh cranial nerves.

The dorsal branch of the vagus nerve originates on the floor of the fourth ventricle near the back of the brainstem. (A ventricle is not a physical structure but a space between the lobes of the brain, filled with cerebrospinal fluid. There are four of these ventricles, interconnected with each other via small canals.)

Both branches of the vagus nerve, along with the ninth and eleventh cranial nerves and the jugular vein, pass through the jugular foramen, a small opening in the base of the skull between the temporal and occipital bones.

Fibers of both the ninth and eleventh cranial nerves weave themselves into the fibers of the tenth cranial nerve. My anatomy teacher, Professor Pat Coughlin, told our class that in modern interpretations of anatomy, an increasing number of teachers consider CN IX and CN X to be two parts of the same nerve. Just as the fibers of the nerves are woven together, their functionality seems to be interrelated as components of the social engagement nervous system.

For clinical purposes of bringing the nervous system into a state of social engagement, I find it simplest to approach the ninth, tenth, and eleventh cranial nerves as if they were one nerve. When a patient presents symptoms indicating a dysfunction in one, there is almost always a dysfunction in the other two. If, after treatment, the patient shows improvement in the test for vagal (CN X) function, the symptoms attributed to dysfunction of the ninth and eleventh cranial nerves usually disappear as well.

MORE ON THE NINTH CRANIAL NERVE

The ninth cranial nerve is called the glossopharyngeal nerve (*glosso-* refers to the tongue, and *pharyngeal* to the pharynx, the back of the top of the throat). This nerve has both afferent (sensory) and efferent (motor) fibers. The efferent branch innervates a single muscle, the stylopharyngeus, which is involved in swallowing.

The ninth cranial nerve receives sensory information from the tonsils, the pharynx, the middle ear, and the posterior third of the tongue. It is also part of the mechanism for regulating blood pressure: it has afferent branches in the carotid sinus, located in the base of the neck near the carotid arteries, and its sensory fibers monitor blood pressure in order to influence the heart and the tonus of the muscle cells in the arteries.

This nerve also monitors oxygen and carbon dioxide levels in the blood, to adjust the breathing rate. It is also responsible for stimulating secretion from the parotid gland, the large salivary gland in front of the ear.

THE TENTH CRANIAL NERVE (THE VAGUS)

The tenth cranial nerve is a vital part of the autonomic nervous system. Before Stephen Porges presented the Polyvagal Theory, the vagus was assumed to function as a single neural pathway. However, we now know that the two branches of the vagus nerve—ventral and dorsal—arise at different places and have very different functions, and this book was written to elucidate those differences and their implications.

An understanding of the two pathways of the vagus nerve provides treatment options for a wide variety of health conditions, discussed later in this book.

THE SUB-DIAPHRAGMATIC (DORSAL) VAGUS BRANCH

The dorsal branch of the vagus nerve has motor fibers that innervate the visceral organs below the respiratory diaphragm: the stomach, liver, spleen, kidneys, gall bladder, urinary bladder, small intestine, pancreas, and the ascending and transverse segments of the colon. Therefore, this branch has sometimes been called the "sub-diaphragmatic branch of the vagus nerve."

However, this description is only partly accurate, since some fibers originating in the dorsal motor nucleus in the brainstem also affect the heart and the lungs, which lie above the diaphragm. Similarly, although the ventral vagus primarily provides motor pathways to the organs above the diaphragm, some fibers influence organs below the diaphragm. All three parts of the autonomic nervous system—the dorsal and ventral branches of the vagus nerve, and the spinal sympathetic chain—affect the vital functions of breathing and blood circulation. Each of the three circuits affects the heart and lungs in different ways.

The Appendix includes two drawings of the visceral organs. (See "Ventral vagus" and "Dorsal vagus.") One shows those innervated by the ventral vagus, and the other shows those innervated by the dorsal vagus.

OTHER FUNCTIONS OF THE VENTRAL BRANCH
OF THE VAGUS NERVE

The ventral branch of the vagus nerve originates in the brainstem, at the top of the spinal cord under the brain. (See "Brain" in the Appendix.) It stimulates rhythmic constriction of the bronchioles, facilitating the extraction of oxygen, while the brainstem area controlling dorsal vagal activation may result in chronic constriction of the airways, making it difficult for air to get through. (This is part of the mechanism that is activated in a state of shutdown or shock. This narrowing of the bronchioles also occurs in COPD, chronic bronchitis, and asthma.)

When we feel safe, the ventral branch of the vagus nerve supports rest or calm activity. There is a rhythmic vacillation of the opening of the airways; they are moderately open on the inbreath and moderately closed on the outbreath.

The ventral branch of the vagus nerve innervates many of the small muscles in the throat, including the vocal cords, larynx, pharynx, and some muscles at the back of the pharynx (the *levator veli palatini* and uvular muscles).

THE ELEVENTH CRANIAL NERVE

The eleventh cranial nerve, or "accessory nerve," is one of the keys to the well-being of the entire musculoskeletal system. Because it innervates the trapezius and sternocleidomastoid (SCM) muscles, which enable the movement of the head and neck, tension in either of these muscles on one side pulls the shoulder, spine, and entire body out of alignment.

Both the trapezius and the sternocleidomastoid muscles originate on the bones of the cranium. (The trapezius attaches to the mastoid process of the temporal bone, and the sternocleidomastoid to the occipital bone.) Together they make up the outer ring of muscles in the neck, shoulders, and upper back.

If the eleventh cranial nerve is dysfunctional, it results in a lack of proper tonus in these muscles. This in turn can cause acute or chronic shoulder problems, stiff neck, migraines, and difficulties rotating the head from side to side. (See Chapter 5 for more information about these muscles. Part Two also contains a treatment for relieving migraines by reducing excessive tensions in these muscles.)

Rather than simply massaging a chronically tense or flaccid trapezius or SCM muscle, it is better for a therapist to first improve the function of the eleventh cranial nerve using the Basic Exercise (see Part Two), and then massage the muscles after the nerve is functional again.

Treating the Cranial Nerves

We need different techniques to treat the cranial nerves than those generally used to treat spinal nerves. To treat spinal-nerve dysfunction some therapists use chiropractics or chiropractic-like mobilizations (short, high-velocity thrusts). A physical therapist may stretch and strengthen the muscles of the neck and back in order to reposition the vertebrae, thereby reducing pressure on spinal nerves. If these modalities fail, we sometimes resort to orthopedic surgery.

However, if we want to manually improve or restore function in the cranial nerves, we need a different approach. Since 1920, there has been a form of treatment for addressing dysfunctions of the cranial nerves, called "cranial osteopathy," "craniosacral therapy (CST)," or "osteopathy in the cranial field (OCF)."

In the United States, doctors of osteopathy (DOs) have the same training as medical doctors. Like their MD counterparts, they are licensed to perform surgical operations, write prescriptions, and work in psychiatric hospitals. An important difference between osteopaths and MDs is that osteopaths have additional training in hands-on treatment techniques.

William Garner Sutherland, DO (1873–1954) founded cranial osteopathy. His student and colleague Harold Magoun, DO (1927–2011), wrote the seminal book *Osteopathy in the Cranial Field,*[8] which was first published in 1951 and is still used today by osteopathic physicians who elect to learn the cranial techniques. Magoun's book describes three approaches to cranial work. One is biomechanical, in which the therapist holds two adjacent cranial bones for the purpose of mobilizing them in the sutures (where two or more skull bones come together). This can reduce mechanical pressure on the cranial nerves where they come through the various openings in the skull.

The biomechanical approach demands a detailed study of cranial anatomy as well as extensive hands-on experience to get the feel of the work and use the techniques effectively. The French osteopath Alain Gehin further developed the system of biomechanical techniques as described by Sutherland and Magoun, and he has taught his approach to students in many countries.

Another cranial treatment approach involves stretching the soft-tissue membranes within the skull and spine. The *dura mater* is a tube of connective tissue extending from the skull to the tailbone and containing the brain, spinal cord, and cerebrospinal fluid. The *falx cerebri* and the *tentorium* are connective-tissue sheets that hold the bones of the skull together and are collectively referred to as the "dural membranes."

All of these dural structures become less flexible with aging, illness, certain kinds of antibiotics, and physical trauma. Harold Magoun described these membranes and how to release tension in them. Later, this work was developed further by John Upledger, DO, and is now taught worldwide by the Florida-based Upledger Institute. His approach includes stretching the dural membranes as well as allowing them to "unwind."

The third approach is called biodynamic craniosacral therapy. Its goal is maximizing movement of the cerebrospinal fluid that circulates around the brain and spinal cord, bringing nourishment to the tissues and helping to eliminate metabolic waste products.

Biodynamic techniques facilitate release by using the flow of the cerebrospinal fluid contained within the dural membranes of the skull and spine. The therapist holds the client's head with an extremely light touch, combined with a keen awareness of the tiny, subtle movements of the cranial bones.[9]

The Spinal Nerves

Most people have heard about problems arising from dysfunctions of the spinal nerves. Many people suffer from a herniated disk that presses on the spinal cord, or a bone growth (spinal stenosis) that can press on a spinal nerve and cause pain, loss of sensation, or loss of function (for example, bladder control). Spinal nerve dysfunction can also cause local paralysis (inability to use a specific skeletal muscle).

Some people use chiropractic or osteopathic treatments to alleviate spinal-nerve compression. Chiropractors usually use high-velocity, short-thrust techniques intended to reposition a vertebra, bringing it into better alignment and taking pressure off of the pain-causing nerve. Osteopaths have the same goal but usually use a more gentle approach.

Other popular "conservative" treatments for the spine include yoga and stretching, strengthening the back muscles with calisthenics, weight training, physical therapy, and massage to balance the tonus of the back muscles. If these methods fail to keep the spine in shape, we may feel invalidated, despondent, and inclined to choose radical treatments such as surgery.

Back surgery is a booming business. About 500,000 Americans undergo surgery each year for lower-back problems alone. According to the US Agency for Health care Research and Quality, we spent more than $30.7 billion in 2008 alone on hospital procedures for back pain.[10] Unfortunately, surgery doesn't always buy relief. And studies show that most backaches go away by themselves in time. The hospital in my town in Denmark has stopped using surgery for back pain.

For decades, orthopedic surgeons have treated back problems by cutting away part of a bulging disk, chiseling away a bone spur, or even inserting a metal plate and screws to stiffen adjacent vertebrae. In spite of the widespread use of surgery, the effectiveness of such operations is not scientifically documented. On the contrary, there is a growing body of research showing that such operations are not effective in the long run.[11,12,13]

One important function of the spinal nerves is to allow us to use our arms, legs, and trunk to move our body by contracting and relaxing various muscles. Spinal nerves also innervate some of the visceral organs. Messages to the spinal nerves originate in the brain and travel through the spinal cord, a tube-like nerve bundle that exits the cranium through a large opening in the base of the skull called the *foramen magnum* (Latin for "large hole").

After exiting the cranium, pairs of spinal nerves emanate from the spinal cord, emerging through spaces between adjacent vertebrae to serve the muscles, joints, ligaments, tendons, internal organs, and skin. Human beings have thirty-three pairs of spinal nerves, with one nerve of each pair going to the right side of the body and the other to the left.

Each pair of spinal nerves corresponds to a segment of the vertebral column. There are thirty-three vertebrae in all: seven in the neck, twelve in the chest, five in the lumbar region, five in the sacrum, and four in the tailbone. The spinal nerves, which include both motor and sensory nerves, carry signals back and forth between the brain and rest of the body. Two important exceptions are the trapezius and the sternocleidomastoid muscles in the neck and shoulder, which receive their innervation from the eleventh cranial nerve; implications of this are discussed elsewhere in this book, including Chapter 5.

There is always more than one branch of one spinal nerve going to any given muscle. This provides insurance that, if one of the spinal nerves is damaged, the muscle can still function (albeit less efficiently) using the signals from other available nerves.

Every spinal nerve also affects several muscles. Often the muscles are part of a chain of movement—for example, muscles in the shoulder, upper arm, forearm, wrist, and fingers work together as a unit to control the basic movements of the arm or hand.

The motor pathways of a nerve signal a muscle to contract. The spinal sensory nerves gather various kinds of information from the body and feed it back to the brain: they carry sensations of pain, positions of the body parts in relationship to each other, movement, tension in the muscles or fascia, and the sense of touch for all of the body except the face (which is innervated by cranial nerves).

Branches of the spinal and cranial nerves are traditionally categorized into motor and sensory functions, but this is an oversimplification. If we look more closely at the individual "motor nerves," we observe that some of their fibers are motor fibers—but that they also contain sensory fibers that report the state of tension in a muscle back to the brain. We now know that the majority of fibers in "motor nerves" are actually sensory.

This combination of sensory and motor nerve fibers provides a feedback loop that allows us to use the motor fibers to tense a muscle while sensory fibers simultaneously send information back to the brain regarding the changing level of tension in the muscle. This allows us to calibrate the tensing of the muscle—a much more powerful and efficient approach than if the muscle could only tense fully or not at all, which would be the case if we had no sensory-fiber feedback.

Under normal conditions, the spinal nerves facilitate easy, well-coordinated, graceful movements, and the muscles fire using the minimum amount of energy to achieve the desired movement. However, if the body is in a state of stress and all the muscles are more tense than necessary, this natural coordination is often lost, and movements become uncoordinated, awkward, or weak.

THE SPINAL SYMPATHETIC CHAIN

Branches of the spinal nerves go to specific bodily structures: the skin (dermatomes), the muscles (myotomes), the visceral organs (viscerotomes), and the ligaments, fascia, and connective tissue (fasciatomes). Rather than a single spinal nerve innervating only one muscle, there is some overlap, so that branches of several spinal nerves may innervate the same individual muscle. This creates a backup system so that if one part of a nerve is damaged, other parts can still contract the same muscle, and it can still function, though it works less efficiently.

Some of the spinal nerves go to the internal organs. For example, the nerves from thoracic vertebrae T1 and T4 go to the heart, the nerves from T5 and T8 go to the lungs, T9 goes to the stomach, and T10 goes to the kidneys. Other nerves serve other structures including the bladder, genital organs, and intestines.

Upon exiting the spinal cord, some thoracic and upper-lumbar spinal nerve fibers (T1–L2) extend laterally a short distance. While some of these stay in the same area, others join fibers from vertebrae above and below to form part of the sympathetic chain. The sympathetic chain extends the length of the vertebral column between T1 and L2, connecting to these spinal nerves. Most of the sympathetics, which project to visceral organs and to the head, are accompanied by arteries to their destinations.

When we face a threat to our survival, there is a surge in the activity of the entire sympathetic chain, spreading the fight-or-flight response to mobilize the resources of the entire body. This response is immediate and total, which is appropriate if we are threatened or in danger. The muscles tense to prepare for movements needed to fight or flee; this is described in weight-lifting circles as getting "pumped up."

Some organs innervated by these sympathetic nerve fibers increase their level of activity in order to support this mobilization. For example, the heart beats faster to supply more blood to the muscular system. The blood pressure increases to be able to pump more blood into tense muscles. The liver releases stored-up sugars into the blood to make extra energy available for the muscles to burn. The survival stress response from the sympathetic chain causes the muscles of the airways to open to the maximum, improving our breathing capacity and taking in the maximum amount of oxygen in order to be fully mobilized to fight or run.

At the same time, other organs (primarily those involved in digestion) are slowed or stopped. There is a loss of appetite, the movement of food in the intestine slows or stops, and the person might experience a sensation of "butterflies" in her stomach.

In cases of threat or challenge, the stress state created by the sympathetic response affects the whole body, and it can involve the muscles of all the segments simultaneously. Activation of the spinal sympathetic chain in the "fight or flight" response is one of the three possible states of the autonomic nervous system, to be discussed in more detail later.

The Enteric Nervous System

The enteric nervous system is a network of nerves interconnecting the visceral organs. We know next to nothing about these nerves; because they are so interwoven with each other, with the visceral organs, and with the connective tissue between the organs, it has been impossible so far for anatomists to fully trace the pathways of the enteric nerves. Therefore, we do not find them well represented in most anatomy books.

Furthermore, we know almost nothing of how the enteric nerves function. At best we can guess that the enteric nerves in some way help the different visceral organs to communicate with each other in order to coordinate the very complex process of digestion.

The enteric nervous system is even sometimes referred to as "the second brain," possessing an intelligence that operates beyond our conscious awareness.[14] We can neither consciously know what is going on in our digestive process nor regulate it voluntarily.

CHAPTER 2

The Polyvagal Theory

Whether you can observe a thing or not depends on the theory you use. It is the theory that decides what can be observed.

—Albert Einstein

The Three Circuits of the Autonomic Nervous System

Traditionally the autonomic nervous system was recognized for its regulation of the various visceral "automatic" functions, such as digestion, respiration, sex drive, reproduction, etc. The old model of stress-or-relaxation was based on recognizing only two circuits—the sympathetic and the parasympathetic.

In the old model, the sympathetic nervous system was seen as active in stress response to threats and danger. The parasympathetic nervous system, by contrast, expressed itself in the relaxation response and was associated with the function of the vagus nerve. This older, almost universally accepted model of the autonomic nervous system assumed that there is a single vagus nerve, and it did not take account of the fact that there are actually two quite different neural pathways that are both called "vagus."

The Polyvagal Theory begins by recognizing that the vagus nerve has two separate branches—two separate, distinct vagal nerves that originate in two different locations. We get a more accurate representation of the workings of the autonomic nervous system if we consider that the autonomic nervous system consists of three neural circuits: the ventral branch of the vagus nerve (positive states of relaxation and social engagement), the spinal sympathetic chain (fight or flight), and the dorsal branch of the vagus nerve (slowdown, shutdown, and depressive behavior). These three circuits regulate our bodily functions in order to help us maintain homeostasis.

The Polyvagal Theory also presents another dimension to our understanding of the autonomic nervous system. The autonomic nervous system not only regulates the function of our inner organs; these three circuits also relate to our emotional states, which in turn drive our behavior.

People who give massage know from experience that one person's body might be too tight, another might be too soft, and a third can feel "just right." Usually, when therapists are trained to give massage, they learn to release tension in a tense muscle. However, this approach does not work on a body that lacks sufficient tone.

Goldilocks and the Three ANS States

A good metaphor for the three states of the autonomic nervous system can be found in the fairy tale "Goldilocks and the Three Bears."

Goldilocks was wandering alone in the woods when she came to the cabin belonging to the three bears. She knocked on the door, but no one answered. Being tired and hungry, she decided to go inside and wait until someone returned.

Goldilocks noticed three bowls of porridge on the table. When she tasted them, she found that the first was too hot, the next was too cool, and the third was just right.

After she ate that third bowl of porridge, she saw three beds and decided to take a nap. The first bed was too hard, and the second too soft—but the third one was just right, so she lay down on that one and fell asleep, contented.

The quality of the tone of the musculature in the three autonomic states can be described as one of the following: too hard or hot (in the fight or flight state of spinal sympathetic activity), too soft or cold (in the shutdown state of dorsal vagal activity), and just right (in the state of social engagement, based on the activity of the ventral branch of the vagus and the other four cranial nerves related to social engagement).

Activity supported by the spinal sympathetic chain enables us to fight in order to meet a threat, or run away in order to avoid it. This is because hard, tense muscles allow us to move the entire body more quickly. Higher blood pressure is also needed to get the flow of blood into muscles that are tensed and hard.

Low levels of muscle tonus are found when the dorsal vagal circuit is activated, when there is no need to tense the muscles to fight or flee (or, in some cases of extreme danger, when the body's survival response is to shut down). Low blood pressure is sufficient to get the blood into soft, limp muscles. In its extreme form, this low blood pressure may cause people to lose consciousness and faint. The medical term for this is "syncope."

Normal blood pressure is appropriate for muscles that are neither tense nor flaccid—muscles that feel just right. In states of social engagement, there is generally no threat or danger in our environment or body. Our nervous system registers this fact, so we do not have to do anything; we can truly relax and enjoy being with others. In terms of the Polyvagal Theory, we can be immobilized without fear, anger, or depressive activity when we are in a state of social engagement. Our blood pressure, blood sugar, and temperature are all normal. We can be still, yet awake and alert.

A handshake gives us a good indication of the state of another person's autonomic nervous system. An overly tight body usually results from a chronic state of activity in the spinal sympathetic chain, where the entire muscular system is continually prepared to fight or flee. Such a person characteristically has an overly forceful handshake, squeezing harder than necessary. The opposite is true for someone lacking muscular tonus—usually a sign of overactivity in the dorsal vagal circuit. This person generally has a limp, damp, and sometimes cold handshake.

If our handshake is just right, it is the ventral branch of the vagus nerve that is predominant. We may have some tensions in individual muscles, but the tense muscles relax very quickly, and a massage therapist will notice that our body also feels right.

The tonus of the muscles is only one of many ways to monitor the state of the body's nervous system.

HOMEOSTASIS AND THE ANS

The neural circuits controlling the nerves regulating visceral-organ function can be compared to a thermostat linked to both a heater and an air conditioner. When the thermostat registers that the air is too cold, it turns on the heater, and if the air is too warm, it turns on the air conditioner. Mammals similarly need to maintain body temperature within upper and lower limits, and their sensory nerves provide feedback about body temperature to their "thermostat."

Behavioral patterns as well as physiological functions help the body to regulate temperature. For example, if we are cold, we can move around to produce heat through the activity of our muscles, or we can put on more clothes to insulate ourselves and reduce the loss of body heat. The blood vessels of the skin constrict to conserve heat. When we are very cold, our bodies start to shiver uncontrollably, producing heat from the action of the muscles.

When we are warm, we lie down or sit still in order to reduce muscular activity and thereby avoid further overheating. The blood vessels dilate, allowing more heat to reach the skin surface where it can be dissipated. We take off layers of clothing, and we sweat; when our sweat evaporates, it cools the body.

When people are angry, we sometimes say that they are "hot under the collar." We might admonish them to "cool it." When people do not like something, they may withdraw, and we say that they are "cool" to it. We think of ways to "warm them up" to the idea. Both heat and coolness are sensed as reflections of emotional states.

The three parts of the autonomic nervous system work together to control the activity of the organs, bring about homeostasis, and help us continue to appropriately meet environmental situations and balance conditions within the body.

We can also apply the model of the Polyvagal Theory to problems and diagnoses in many physiological areas such as digestion or reproduction, which we might otherwise consider to be physical issues beyond our control or influence.

For example, there is a growing body of scientific research that uses heart rate variability (HRV) to measure ventral vagal activity by quantifying a spontaneous rhythm in heart rate known as respiratory sinus arrhythmia. These studies find that low levels of ventral vagal activity are linked to a wide range of health issues, such as obesity, high blood pressure, heart fluctuations, etc.[15] There are also some speculations that HRV is a potentially useful measurement to help predict the onset of cancer, cancer metastasis, or the likely mortality of people with cancer.[16] (For more about HRV, see Chapter 4.)

The Five States of the Autonomic Nervous System

BIOBEHAVIOR: THE INTERACTION OF BEHAVIOR AND BIOLOGICAL PROCESSES

Unlike the old model of the autonomic nervous system, which focused exclusively on its regulation of the function of the visceral organs, the new model of the autonomic nervous system includes three distinct neural pathways, as described above, and relates each of these three neural circuits with an emotional state, which drives our behavior. In addition to these three states, we have two hybrid states, each of which combines two of the individual circuits, for a total of five possible conditions of our autonomic nervous system.

One hybrid state supports the experience of intimacy: the dorsal vagus is engaged to slow down our physical activity, at the same time as the ventral vagus allows a feeling of safety with another person. This is discussed in further detail below.

The second hybrid state expresses itself in friendly competition. We may fight extremely hard to win in sports or games, but this occurs within a framework of safety and rules to which all of the opponents have agreed in advance. In this hybrid state, the fight or flight response of spinal sympathetic chain activation is combined with the feelings of safety associated with activity of the ventral vagus branch.

THE THREE NEURAL PATHWAYS OF THE ANS

The first of the autonomic nervous system's neural pathways is the social-engagement nervous system. It involves activity in the ventral branch of the vagus nerve (CN X) and four other cranial nerves (CN V, VII, IX, and XI). Activity in this circuit has a calming, soothing effect, and promotes rest and restitution.

The ventral branch of the vagus nerve relates to positive emotions of joy, satisfaction, and love. In terms of behavior, it expresses itself in positive social activities with friends and loved ones. The state of social engagement supports social behaviors in which we support and share with other people. Cooperation with others usually improve our chances for survival—we talk together, sing together, dance together, share a meal, cooperate to complete a project, teach and nurture children, etc.

The second of the ANS's neural pathways is the spinal sympathetic chain, which is activated when our survival is threatened. If we mobilize our body with this response, we can make an extra effort to help us respond to the threat. This state of "mobilization with fear" arises when we are not safe, or do not feel safe. The spinal sympathetic chain relates to emotions of anger or fear, which can express themselves in behaviors such as fighting in order to overcome the threat or fleeing to avoid a threatening situation.

The third neural pathway is the dorsal branch of the vagus nerve. This pathway is activated when we face an overwhelming force and imminent destruction. When there is no point in fighting or running away, we conserve what resources we have—we immobilize. Activation of this pathway fosters feelings of helplessness, hopelessness, and apathy, manifesting in withdrawal and shutdown. This state can be described as "immobilization with fear."

When humans or other mammals are faced with seemingly inevitable mortal danger, death, or destruction, the dorsal branch of our vagus nerve is activated. A sudden or extreme surge of dorsal vagal activity can give rise to a state of shock, or shutdown. Among other responses, the muscular system loses its tonus, and the blood pressure drops. We might faint or go into a state of shock (syncope).

Wildlife documentaries on the African plains have captured the following scene. A lion chases and captures a baby antelope, and takes it up in its mighty jaws. The baby antelope had been in a state of spinal sympathetic chain activity when it was threatened and ran away. Now, facing imminent death, it goes into shock and shutdown: it faints, and its body goes limp.

Lions are not generally scavengers. If a lion suddenly senses that that its prey has become lifeless, it may open its jaws, drop the prey, and move away. Just when the lion is about to shake the baby antelope in order to break its neck, or to sink its teeth into its flesh, the limp muscles fail to give the usual resistance. Perhaps the antelope's shutdown response is enough to nullify the lion's killer instinct. The lion releases its grip, the baby antelope falls to the ground, and the lion moves away.

A few seconds after the lion leaves, the baby antelope stands up, shakes it off, and returns to its mother. It then resumes grazing as if nothing has happened. The baby antelope is ready to face the next challenge to its survival, thanks to its life-saving shutdown response. This illustrates the adaptive survival value of the dorsal-branch immobilization response in situations of extreme danger.

We see another example of how the dorsal branch of the vagus nerve can facilitate a successful defense: A porcupine, facing danger from a predator, withdraws by rolling up into a ball. Its sharp quills bristle outward, making it impossible for the predator to successfully bite it.

THE TWO HYBRID CIRCUITS

In addition to these three circuits of the autonomic nervous system, there are two hybrid states made up of different combinations of two of the three neural circuits.

The fourth state is a hybrid that supports friendly competition, or "mobilization without fear," which is appropriate when we engage in competitive sports. This state combines the effects of two neural circuits: activation of the spinal sympathetic chain allows us to mobilize ourselves in order to achieve our best performance. Activation of the social engagement circuit keeps things friendly, so that we can play safely within the rules and avoid hurting each other.

In sports, we can fight very hard to win. Both teams agree to follow the rules and stay within boundaries to keep everything safe. After all, it is only a game. There are many other examples of mobilization without fear. Puppies from the same litter constantly play with each other as if they were fighting. They growl and they bite each other for hours on end.

In Japan, lovers sometimes have a ritual pillow fight. The pillows are overfilled with feathers, and slit open along one side. Within a few hits, the feathers come out of the pillowcase and fly around until they have filled the whole room, usually to the great amusement of the lovers. What started out as a "fight" now elicits smiles and laughs from both of them.

The fifth state is also a hybrid of two neural circuits. Activity in the dorsal branch of the vagus nerve, when combined with that of the ventral branch of the vagus nerve, supports feelings of intimacy and intimate behavior. This state, which we could call "immobilization without fear," is characterized by calm, trusting feelings, allowing us, for example, to lie still and cuddle with a loved one.

The Vagus Nerve

Physical well-being and emotional well-being are intimately linked. If we have a headache, it can be difficult to be happy, joyful, and interested in connecting with other people. On the other hand, when we have had a sound night's sleep, some exercise, and a good meal, we feel on top of things and naturally want to be sociable. This connection is well known.

However, not many of us know that a nerve called the vagus helps regulate most of the bodily functions necessary for our health and emotional well-being. This nerve must function properly in order for us to be healthy, feel good emotionally, and interact positively with family, friends, and others.

HISTORICAL RECOGNITION OF THE VAGUS NERVE

The *anatomy* of the nervous system describes where the nerves are located in the body in relationship to muscles, bones, skin, visceral organs, etc. The *physiology* of the nervous system describes the function of these nerves—how they monitor what is going on at different places in the body, how they gather and integrate this information, and how they send signals to control various body functions.

A thorough study of the anatomy and physiology of the nervous system is a major undertaking. Together, anatomy and physiology have formed the foundation of knowledge taught in the first half of the medical school curriculum. For at least the past century, the study of these two disciplines has also found its way into the education of almost all other health care professionals in the Western world.

The first recorded mention of the vagus nerve came from the Greek physician Claudius Galen (130–200 AD), who lived in the Roman Empire and studied the vagus nerve in gladiators whose injuries he treated, and also in the Barbary apes and pigs that he dissected in order to learn more about the body. Galen noted certain dysfunctions that occurred when the vagus nerve had been severed in some of the gladiators.

Galen's writings on the vagus nerve were only part of his legacy. In fact, his writings comprise half of all writings on any subject that have survived from ancient Greece. His vast writings were so widespread and respected that they served as the foundation of European medicine for more than 1,500 years. Since Galen's first explorations, the vagus nerve has been included in all medical texts as well as in papers and books by many psychologists.

Over the centuries, as medical doctors and other health care professionals built upon Galen's observations, they came to believe that the autonomic nervous system consisted of two divisions, the sympathetic and the parasympathetic, both of which innervate the visceral organs. According to this interpretation, the sympathetic division is activated in states of stress, and helps to mobilize the body to fight or flee—or freeze, if need be. The parasympathetic nervous system was understood to consist primarily of the vagus nerve, and to promote relaxation, rest, and restitution,

The almost universally accepted idea was that the sympathetic and parasympathetic nervous systems comprise a balanced system, adjusting their activity accordingly as a person moves back and forth between states of stress and relaxation. The old idea of the autonomic nervous system can be likened to two children on a seesaw: when one child goes down, the child on the other side goes up, and vice versa.

For the last century or so, chronic stress has been identified as a health problem involved in heart disease, asthma, diabetes, and a host of other illnesses. Therefore, relaxation deriving from a well-functioning vagus nerve was considered to be essential to health. The vagus nerve was thought to ensure proper function of the visceral organs responsible for circulation (heart and spleen), respiration (bronchioles and lungs), digestion (stomach, pancreas, liver, gall bladder, and small intestine), and elimination (the ascending and transverse parts of the large intestine, and the kidneys and ureters).

In addition to the vagus nerve, a definition of the "relaxed state" usually included activity of the sacral parasympathetic pathways that go to the descending colon, rectum, bladder, and lower portions of the ureters. Some of these pathways also innervate the genitalia, enabling various sexual reactions. Part of the "parasympathetics" included sacral nerves that come from the sacrum at the base of the spine. Taken together with the vagus nerve, these were characterized as the "rest and digest" or "feed and breed" system.

In 1994, in his presidential lecture for the Society for Psychophysiological Research, Stephen Porges introduced his Polyvagal Theory, which he built around a new understanding of the function of the vagus nerve. A year later, he published these ideas in the journal *Psychophysiology*[17] in an article entitled "Orienting in a Defensive World: Mammalian Modifications of our Evolutionary Heritage—A Polyvagal Theory."

Porges presented a radically different model of the autonomic system. Whereas his concept of stress is similar to the older model, he focused on three divisions of the autonomic nervous system: the ventral branch of the vagus nerve, the sympathetic nervous system, and the dorsal branch of the vagus nerve.

Two Branches of the Nerve Called "Vagus"

The dorsal and ventral branches of the vagus nerve (CN X) originate at different locations in the brain and brainstem, have different pathways through the body, and have very different functions. There is actually no direct anatomical or functional connection between the two; they are separate and distinct entities.

Before the Polyvagal Theory, we did not adequately differentiate between these two branches of the vagus nerve. The ventral branch was lumped together with the dorsal under the heading "the vagus nerve" or "tenth cranial nerve." This has caused longstanding confusion in our attempts to understand the function of the autonomic nervous system.

The Polyvagal Theory makes it possible to appreciate the differences between the two branches of the vagus nerve. The ventral and dorsal branches arise at different locations; the word *ventral* refers to the location of the ventral branch of the vagus nerve, which originates in the *nucleus ambiguus* on the ventral (front, or stomach) side of the brainstem. The word *dorsal* means "toward the back"; as mentioned earlier, the dorsal vagus arises in the floor of the fourth ventricle. The two branches of the vagus nerve evoke very different physiological states, affect the individual visceral organs differently, support different emotional responses, and promote different behaviors. The ventral branch of the vagus nerve functions in conjunction with four other cranial nerves (V, VII, IX, and XI), which also originate in the brainstem. The ventral vagus is myelinated, i.e., insulated by a covering of Schwann cells (connective-tissue cells) that enable it to transmit information more rapidly than non-myelinated nerves. The dorsal vagus, the older of the two, is not myelinated.

In contrast to the sympathetic nervous system, which enables extreme mobilization to facilitate fight or flight, the two branches of the vagus nerve can both bring about immobilization. However, the ventral vagus and the dorsal vagus produce two very different states of immobilization, based on two very different kinds of physiological activity; they are associated with two different types of behavior, evoke two different emotional responses, and have different effects on the visceral organs.

EFFECTS OF ACTIVITY IN THE VENTRAL VAGUS CIRCUIT

When the ventral branch of the vagus nerve and the associated four cranial nerves function properly, human beings and other mammals enjoy the desirable state of social engagement. To be socially engaged, we need to feel safe, with no need to overcome or avoid any external threat by fighting or fleeing; we also need to be physically healthy. When we are socially engaged, we do not need to do anything, or to change anything; we can afford to be immobilized without fear (relaxed). We can maintain a vibrant tone without being collapsed or overly aroused.

The ventral branch of the vagus nerve, together with the other four associated cranial nerves, promotes rest and restitution, ensuring that the physiological prerequisites are present for optimal physical and emotional health, friendship, cooperation, mutual support, parent-child bonding, and loving relationships. When we are socially engaged, we can be creative, positive, productive, and happy.

Sometimes the ventral vagus is called the "new vagus" because it is more recent in terms of its appearance in our phylogenetic species history than the dorsal vagus. The ventral branch is newer in terms of evolution; it is found only in mammals, and in no other class of vertebrates, though there is the possibility that birds may have an equivalent to a ventral vagal pathway. According to Stephen Porges, the two branches of the vagus nerve emerged at different stages in the evolutionary development of vertebrates.

When we (or other mammals) are safe in our environment—free from threats, danger, and unnecessary worries—and in good physical health, we normally exhibit behavior that is socially engaged.

When we are threatened or in danger, however, our autonomic nervous system shuts down the activity of the ventral branch of the vagus nerve and regresses to an earlier, more primitive evolutionary response of either spinal sympathetic activity (flight/fight) or depressive behavior (withdrawal).

If we have a well-functioning nervous system and are socially engaged, we might naturally meet a new situation with openness, trust, and positive expectations. We feel safe, and might first try to communicate, cooperate, and share. Even in the face of a threat, our behavior might still be open and friendly at first. Sometimes this positive, prosocial behavior can also make the other person feel safe, which in turn might be enough to defuse a potentially threatening situation.

However, if this prosocial behavior is not enough to neutralize the threat or danger, our evolutionarily most recent neural mechanism— the social engagement circuit—is the first to be abandoned. We leave the realm of rational thought and conscious choice, and all of our energy goes into instinctive, defensive responses.

If our autonomic nervous system feels that a situation is unsafe, our response can shift down one phylum, from social engagement to the level of reptiles with a strong spinal sympathetic chain response, and we might fight to overcome the threat, or flee to avoid it. If the situation is so extreme that fighting or fleeing is not enough, we may shift down even further and shut down or collapse into a dorsal vagal state of withdrawal, dissociation, and shutdown.

EFFECTS OF ACTIVITY IN THE DORSAL VAGUS CIRCUIT

The dorsal branch is the older of the two branches of the vagus nerve, and is present in all classes of vertebrates, from boneless fish up to and including human beings and other mammals. It is sometimes referred to as the "old vagus."

The Polyvagal Theory describes two autonomic nervous-system states that employ the dorsal vagal circuit. The dorsal vagus, acting on its own, brings about a state of metabolic shutdown. It enables animals to reduce the activity level in their vital functions, thereby conserving energy. This can be described as "immobilization with fear": we are afraid, but we do nothing to confront the danger or run away; we just give up.

The other state involving the dorsal vagal circuit is "immobilization without fear," which combines activity in the dorsal vagal circuit with activity in the social engagement circuit. This state is appropriate when we feel safe and choose to be relatively immobilized in order to be intimate with another person.

The hibernation of mammals involves some degree of dorsal vagal activity, but it is not the same as shutdown. Bears hibernate in winter, for example, but it is more of a slowdown than a shutdown. Bears are warm-blooded and, like all other mammals, need to maintain a minimum oxygen intake and body temperature, often higher than the temperature of the surrounding air, in order to keep their brain functioning and undamaged by hypothermia.

By contrast, reptiles can shutdown almost totally, reducing their heart rate, breathing, and digestion drastically to conserve energy until their next meal. A turtle shuts down its metabolism and life processes as it sleeps in the wintry, near-freezing waters at the bottom of a freshwater pond; its body temperature falls to the temperature of the surrounding water. The turtle is cold-blooded and does not produce its own energy to raise its body temperature. Instead, it will often lie on a rock to gather warmth from the sun and air. The winter hibernation of a bear in its cave involves a lesser degree of dorsal vagus activity, which is quite different from the near-total shutdown of a cold-blooded reptile such as a turtle. The bear's body temperature falls only a few degrees.

A sudden, extreme surge in dorsal vagal activity when we or other mammals are faced with mortal danger can result in a state of shock, or immobilization with fear. Although I sometimes refer to this physiological state as "shutdown," in mammals it is more precise to think of it as a drastic slowdown. This immobilization with fear can be used as a defensive strategy, as in behaviors such as freezing and feigning death. For example, a mouse freezes when it senses a predator nearby, becoming "as still as a mouse" to avoid detection.

Hawks have extremely good eyesight and can pick up the slightest movement, even those of a mouse's normal breathing. If a hawk is circling in a field over a mouse, the hawk will see any mouse that tries to run away and will swoop down and catch it in its sharp claws. So, instead of employing the defense strategy of fleeing, the mouse freezes. It slows down its vital activity and holds its breath until the hawk has flown away and the danger is over.

However, if the slowdown is too sudden or too extreme, it can result in the mouse being literally scared to death. About 10 percent of mice die from shutting down as a response to danger from a bird of prey or a snake.

The Polyvagal Theory describes how a surge in the activity of the dorsal branch of the vagus nerve is a defensive strategy that causes a physiological state of shock or shutdown to help us cope with traumatic events, extreme danger, or imminent destruction, whether real or imagined, by suddenly collapsing and shutting down. Giving up or feigning death can be lifesaving; by not moving, we might avoid the attention of a predator or enemy. Physiologically, immobilization also conserves energy.

However, remaining chronically in a dorsal vagal state when there is no longer any threat or danger robs us of our clarity, productivity, and joy of living until we can get back into a state of social engagement. In our culture, we have become preoccupied with problems stemming from stress. Unfortunately, we have remained largely unaware that another danger to our health arises from the widespread condition of chronic activation of the dorsal vagus circuit.

When dorsal vagal activity is less extreme but chronic, its emotional correlate is characterized by depressive feelings. In everyday conversation, many people say that they experience "depression," or describe their mood and behavior as "depressed," without having been diagnosed as such by a psychiatrist or psychologist. For the purposes of this book, I prefer to use the terms "depressive feelings" and "depressive behavior" or "activity of the dorsal branch of the vagus nerve," and to generally avoid the term depression, which is a medical or psychological diagnosis.

People with a diagnosis of depression, or people in a depressed state, typically lose interest in activities that once were pleasurable. They overeat, experience loss of appetite, or have digestive problems. They have reduced energy, and they become inactive, introverted, apathetic, helpless, and asocial. They can feel sad, anxious, empty, hopeless, worthless, guilty, irritable, ashamed, or restless. They may experience lethargy, lack of energy, and a lack of goal-oriented activity.

They can have problems concentrating, remembering details, or making decisions, and are often plagued by the aches and pains of fibromyalgia. They may contemplate, attempt, or commit suicide. These can all be symptoms of activity in the dorsal branch of the vagus nerve.

The medical literature has generally focused on the physiology of chronic stress, with less attention given to the physiology underlying chronic depression. But when people come to my clinic with a diagnosis of depression from a psychologist or psychiatrist, or when they exhibit depressive behavior, I find that that their problem is usually accompanied by a state of activation of the dorsal branch of their vagus nerve.

If the transition into a dorsal state has involved a sudden surge in dorsal-branch activity, the event can be described as a shock or trauma, and we can describe its effect as "shutdown." When a person faces an overwhelmingly dangerous situation and/or the possibility of imminent death, it is a natural reaction to dissociate from one's own body, from the here and now; to shut down physically, emotionally, and mentally; and perhaps even to faint.

Ideally, when the danger has passed, we should move out of this state and back to social engagement; we should "come back to our senses." However, many people get stuck at some level of this state of immobilization with fear. In this case, it is appropriate to suspect that there is chronic activation of the dorsal vagal circuit.

Prior to the Polyvagal Theory, depression and depressive behaviors issues lacked a physiological model in terms of the nervous system. It neither fit into the category of stress nor that of relaxation. Perhaps this is why it has been so difficult to find safe, non-addictive, and effective treatments for conditions such as depression.

Stephen Porges's Polyvagal Theory focuses on the relationships of the autonomic nervous system, the emotions, and behavior. His work has awakened a growing interest in applications of these understandings by psychologists, psychiatrists, and an array of gifted, insightful trauma therapists. He describes what he calls the "vagal brake"—how activation of the social engagement circuit "puts the brakes on" the other circuits and lifts us out of a chronic dorsal vagal or spinal sympathetic state.

Under normal conditions of challenges to survival, the spinal sympathetic chain or the dorsal branch of the vagal nerve may be triggered into active states of defense. However, when social engagement is coupled with either of these circuits, the range of human behavior is expanded by keeping the individual out of a defensive state. When social engagement joins together with the spinal sympathetic chain, this hybrid enables friendly movements, including symbolic fighting, which are at the heart of the human activity of play. When the dorsal vagal circuit support of immobilization is joined with the protective regulatory features of the ventral vagus and other components of the social engagement system such as prosodic vocalizations, feelings of intimacy may spontaneously emerge. People can be close together physically and share the positive feelings of love.

Using the exercises in this book, it should only take a minute or two to get back into a state of social engagement.

SYMPTOMS OF A DORSAL VAGAL STATE

If we are not socially engaged, we can experience many negative physical and emotional symptoms when faced with adverse conditions. One response is the state of mobilization of the spinal sympathetic chain, characterized by activities of fight or flight.

The other response comes from activation of the dorsal vagal circuit: Our muscles and connective tissues lose their normal tonus, soften, and go limp, and our body feels heavy. To someone else, our muscles feel flaccid. If we try to do even a small task, it takes a monumental effort to move.

In this state we typically feel helpless, apathetic, and hopeless. Our heartbeat slows, and our blood pressure drops; the blood withdraws from the periphery of the body and gathers in the center. Much of the blood, full of oxygen and nutrients that normally would go to the arms and legs to enable a fight-or-flight response in spinal sympathetic chain activity, is retracted to the thorax and abdomen to maintain minimal levels of the basic visceral functions. Thus our hands and feet feel cold and clammy.

When we are in a dorsal vagal state, we often have pains that move around to different places in the body. Most people believe that pain in the body comes from tight muscles, and therapists usually massage the body where it hurts and/or it where muscles are hard. But often, when a massage therapist alleviates pain at one place, another pain arises somewhere else.

This may seem inexplicable to massage therapists who know that they did a good job making a once-hard muscle now feel soft. The client, not acknowledging improvement from what we have done, says, "Now the pain has moved to here." So the therapist chases the pain from one place to another, without the client actually feeling better. This condition is often diagnosed as fibromyalgia.

Rather than simply massaging an area that hurts, the best way to treat this condition is to elevate the person from a dorsal vagal state by activating the ventral circuit state, for example, with the Basic Exercise (see Part Two).

There are other commonly observable signs when we are in a state of shock or shutdown: The face loses its color and appears lifeless and unresponsive; the facial expression is unchanging and facial muscles sag. The voice also lacks prosody (melodic expressiveness); it is flat and without melody. The eyes appear dull and lifeless—there is no sparkle. We may also have low blood pressure, which can cause dizziness or fainting (vasovagal syncope). This occurs because, if our muscles are undertoned, our blood pressure does not need to be high in order to push blood through the lowered resistance in the muscles.

Dorsal vagal state may also be involved in POTS (postural orthostatic tachycardia syndrome). People with POTS typically faint when they stand up and their blood pressure drops. They often exhibit numerous symptoms of autonomic nervous system deregulation. Many POTS symptoms seem to be caused by an imbalance of the autonomic nervous system's control over blood flow and blood pressure. The autonomic nervous system regulates the necessary adjustments in vascular tone, heart rate, and blood pressure when we stand up. In POTS, the system seems to be out of balance, and blood is not going to the right places.[18]

Activation of the dorsal vagus circuit can also cause sweating or nausea. In extreme situations, such as in sudden and severe fright, there can be a loss of bladder and anal-sphincter control. Breathing slows, and the volume of each breath is far less than usual. Our mental awareness turns inward, or even disappears entirely when overwhelming danger presents itself, resulting in dissociation, a withdrawal of consciousness from the body. We are not in the here and now, and we may feel as if we are having an out-of-body experience, as if watching what is going on from a great distance.

The blood flow to the frontal lobes of our brain is also reduced by dorsal vagus activation. These lobes are where our higher functions reside; the frontal lobes are considered the human part of the brain and are involved with the functions of language and will. By "will," I mean conceiving an idea to do something, and monitoring our progress toward that goal.

Often, after a traumatic event, we say that we do not remember what happened. Our brain is incapable of forming verbalizations or visualizations about what had been going on at the time because we were reacting from a different, more primitive part of our brain and nervous system.

Dissociation is a widespread problem. It can be characterized as ongoing activity of the dorsal vagus nerve that keeps us in a physiological state of fear. We may be present in a group but not take part in a conversation; we may be lethargic and lack empathy. We might talk a lot but say nothing meaningful about ourselves or our situation. We cannot set goals or take actions to bring about changes that could help us in life. This depressive mindset is supported by chronic activity of the dorsal branch of the vagus nerve.

However, if we are without fear, dorsal vagal activity has quite a different effect. The state of immobilization without fear, based on dorsal vagal activity combined with the activity of the cranial nerves of social engagement, provides the physiological foundation for rest and restitution, and supports intimacy.

EFFECTS OF VENTRAL VAGUS ACTIVITY

A step above reptiles, at the top of the evolutionary ladder, the class of mammals including human beings has attained a more sophisticated nervous system that includes ventral as well as dorsal vagal circuits. (Note that modern reptiles are not the evolutionary ancestors of mammals; primitive, now-extinct reptiles are our evolutionary precursors.)

In the entire animal kingdom, only mammals have a ventral circuit, which is the ventral branch of the vagus nerve. To activate this ventral vagal circuit, the individual must both be and feel safe in terms of the environment, as well as in terms of feedback from the proprioceptive nerves that monitor what is going on in the body.

The ventral vagal circuit can be active when we are physically active, or when we are immobile. It gives rise to the state of social engagement, together with four other cranial nerves (CN V, VII, IX and XI). Social engagement goes far beyond the simple concept of "relaxation" in the old model of the autonomic nervous system, with its two-state vacillation between stress and relaxation. The ventral vagal state allows us to rest and restore ourselves. We are not in a state of fear, and we can choose to be immobile. We can sit in a rocking chair on the back porch on a warm summer evening with someone we like, and watch the sun go down. We can listen to music. We can daydream or meditate.

When we are not socially engaged, on the other hand, we can experience many negative physical and emotional symptoms such as the state of sympathetic nervous system mobilization, characterized by fight or flight, or dorsal vagal immobilization (frozen and/or with depressed behavior).

Despite these very different functions of the vagal and dorsal branches, it is not surprising that Galen and the anatomists who followed after him were not aware that the dorsal and ventral vagus branches are separate entities. When Galen looked into the wounds of the gladiators, or dissected pigs and Barbary apes, he did not have the luxury we have today in the dissecting rooms of our universities; he could not cool the cadavers, preserve them with formaldehyde, or observe them under microscopes.

Given all these difficulties, it is remarkable that Galen was able to discover so much detail about the anatomy of the vagal nerves, and with such accuracy. Yet his understandable failure to distinguish between the two nerve branches that share the name "vagus" has misled students and practitioners of anatomy, physiology, psychology, and medicine for thousands of years.

Stress and the Sympathetic Nervous System

Just as use of the word "depression" is widespread and often inaccurate, the word "stress" has been so widely used that its meaning has become imprecise. It is more precise to describe stress as the physiological state that arises from activation of the spinal sympathetic nervous system, resulting in a fight-or-flight response.

The old stress/relaxation model considered stress to be the opposite of relaxation. It did not describe what happens to the visceral organs in the physiological state of shock or the related emotional state of depression—both of which express immobilization with fear. Nor was there an appreciation of the separate physical structures in the nervous system that are responsible for shock or depressive feelings on one hand and social engagement on the other.

In the Polyvagal model, the vagus nerve, long thought to be responsible for a single state of relaxation, is now understood to include two distinct pathways that activate two different non-stress states—neither of which exactly corresponds to relaxation in the older model of the autonomic nervous system.

To avoid the confusions that arise from the word "stress," I prefer to use Stephen Porges's description of the fight-or-flight state as "mobilization with fear," and will try to hold to the biological model of stress: the sympathetic nervous system's response (mobilization with fear) to an external event or internal state, maximizing its potential to fight or flee. The neurology underlying this state is major activation of the spinal sympathetic chain. As a defensive strategy, this produces a powerful muscular response with the potential for making an extraordinary effort to save our life (and/or someone else's) in a threatening situation.

Ideally, when the threat passes, activation of the sympathetic chain should also dissipate. If our nervous system is resilient and flexible, our nervous system should naturally return to a state of social engagement. If this does not occur, and activation of the sympathetic chain becomes chronic, it is not good for our physical and emotional health or our social relationships.

Activation of the sympathetic chain is not limited to a defensive strategy. When we are safe and our autonomic nervous system is functioning optimally, there is a slight activation of the sympathetic nervous system on every inbreath, causing our blood pressure to rise and our heart to beat a little faster. The pulse feels a little stronger to the touch. When we breathe out again and this slight sympathetic activation stops, the heart rate and the blood pressure decrease. Our heartbeat should slow down on the outbreath, and our pulse should feel softer.

Therapists can train their fingertip sensitivity to feel this normal change between slight activation of the spinal sympathetic chain and activation of the ventral vagal circuit. If there is no change in the pulse between the inbreath and outbreath, it is a sign of autonomic nervous system dysfunction.

THE FIGHT-OR-FLIGHT RESPONSE

The fight-or-flight response has a number of effects on our physiology, all geared to help us survive in a state of stress when we are threatened. When muscles are tensed, they increase their resistance to blood circulation. In order to pump blood through tense muscles, our blood pressure rises.

Our heart rate also rises, so that we can pump more blood to the muscles. Our bronchioles dilate, helping us breathe more easily, which increases the amount of oxygen reaching our lungs, our blood, and our cells. Better breathing also helps us eliminate more of the waste products of muscle-cell metabolism; we get rid of carbon dioxide (CO_2) on the outbreath. Our liver dumps extra sugar into our bloodstream as a quick source of energy.

Bony fish are the first class of vertebrates with a "spinal" sympathetic nervous system, which is what generates the state biologists call "stress." Amphibians also have a spinal sympathetic nervous system and are also able to flee danger quickly. Reptiles too use their spinal sympathetic state to exert extraordinary physical effort. A crocodile engaging its stress state can move with great speed and power; for short distances, a crocodile can move half again as fast as a champion Olympic sprinter.

This same spinal sympathetic nervous system allows humans and other mammals to use the stress state as a defensive strategy by fighting or running away from a threat (mobilization with fear). Just as for reptiles and amphibians, our states of stress and states of shutdown can provide great flexibility for reacting to various situations.

When used as a defensive strategy, the sympathetic nervous system helps us maximize our ability to fight or to flee. If a person is socially engaged, their sympathetic nervous system can also be temporarily activated in a positive way, along with the social engagement circuits, to facilitate social interchange in play, sporting competition, and even sexual foreplay.

Not limited to the act of physically engaging in violence, the fight response includes the full range of other behaviors aimed at changing things by force: verbal aggression in the form of sarcasm and abuse, passive aggression (opposing by not taking part), random aggression toward strangers, and wanton destruction of property.

Similarly, flight is not only the act of running away—it includes actively avoiding people, situations, or places. It can be simply withdrawing from social situations by watching television or taking part in other solitary activities, possibly driven by anxiety or panic attacks.

Playing violent video games, for instance, might temporarily put our nervous system into a state of arousal and fight, and being addicted to these games and playing them continually might keep us in that state. With this in mind, parents might try to cut down on the time that children sit in front of the computer.

It may also mean that the parents themselves should spend less time in front of their computers. Rather than leaving children alone with the television or electronic devices, it is better for parents to be present with their children, available for social interaction and conversation. Parents should take it upon themselves to initiate play and other social activities with the child and other members of the family—activities that used to come naturally to families before electronics.

A NEW UNDERSTANDING OF STRESS

Although many people talk about being stressed, a large percentage of them are not actually stressed in terms of spinal sympathetic chain activity. Physiologically, some of them are actually in a state of dorsal vagal activity (shutdown or withdrawal); in emotional terms, they are in a depressed state.

This condition can be the result of a traumatic incident sometime in the past. They may have a diagnosis of post-traumatic stress even if they are not physiologically in an actual state of sympathetic-chain stress. According to the Polyvagal Theory, their state is better described as activation of the dorsal branch of the vagus nerve, and these individuals may accordingly suffer from lethargy and immobilization.

The way to move people out of both states—stress with accompanying fight-or-flight behaviors (mobilization with fear) and depressive feelings behaviors with shutdown (immobilization with fear)—is to activate the ventral branch of their vagus nerve.

The three circuits of the autonomic nervous system are hierarchical, with a step-like progression from one state to the next, according to the evolutionary development of the autonomic nervous system in vertebrates. Social engagement, based on the most recently evolved nerve circuit including the ventral vagus branch, is at the top of the ladder, and it promotes peaceful immobilization and a sense of well-being. The next rung down is the spinal sympathetic chain, which activates the fight or flight response. At the bottom, the dorsal vagal circuit, the oldest evolutionary structure, triggers the defensive response of immobilization with fear.

Activity of the ventral branch of the vagus nerve inhibits the two lower levels. Activation of the ventral vagal circuit, supporting activities that are productive in terms of personal survival as well as social activities, lifts us out of chronic activation of the spinal sympathetic system, and it also takes us out of dorsal states of shutdown.

It is not necessary to go up the ladder one step at a time from shutdown to stress and then from stress to social engagement. Ventral vagal circuit activity moves a person directly from shutdown and emotional depression all the way up to a ventral vagal state.

The spinal sympathetic chain is the next rung down. Activity in this circuit inhibits the dorsal vagal circuit. Running, swimming, or other forms of exercise that simulate fight-or-flight exertions often help to bring patients out of depression.[19]

Many types of antidepressant medicine work in a similar fashion. By chemically stressing the body, they temporarily activate the spinal sympathetic chain. However, antidepressant medicine does not bring us up all the way to the level of social engagement, and it can have undesired side effects. Given the choice, I believe that most people would prefer to come out of states of depression by using simple self-help exercises such as those I describe in Part Two.

The goal of my treatments is to bring my clients out of a state of stress or depression and up to the level of social engagement. The exercises and hands-on treatments in this book will, ideally, help many people to achieve a state of social engagement and well-being.

There is good reason for emphasizing the importance of proper function of the ventral branch of the vagus nerve in achieving optimal physical and psychological health. The state of our autonomic nervous system gives us an indication of our general level of physical health and emotional well-being. When our autonomic nervous system is in a state of stress or shutdown, we often have problems with our health, our relationships, and our emotional states. In my clinic and practice, if testing shows the ventral branch of the vagus nerve to be dysfunctional (see Chapter 4), my first goal is to get this nerve to function properly.

Over the years, I have used different techniques to help move people out of stressed or depressed states and restore their ventral vagal branch function. For the last few years, I have found it sufficient to have my clients help themselves by practicing the Basic Exercise (see Part Two).

In some cases (for example, with babies, small children, or individuals on the autism spectrum), it can be difficult or impossible to communicate sufficiently with language to get them to do the exercise properly for themselves. In such cases, I use hands-on techniques from biomechanical craniosacral therapy. A description of one of these can be found in "The Neuro-Fascial Release Technique" (also in Part Two).

After clients do the Basic Exercise, or after I have used my hands-on technique, I test their vagal function again to ascertain whether the desired change has been achieved. After the ventral branch of the vagus nerve has come to proper functionality, I apply additional techniques from biomechanical craniosacral therapy. In many cases, when their ventral vagus has been brought to a proper function, their health issues diminish or disappear.[20]

"But you're not a doctor!" some people may say. No, I am not. In my clinic, I do not make any form of medical diagnosis, or treat disease. Giving a diagnosis and treating disease with prescription drugs fall solely within the responsibility of a well-trained medical doctor. All I can do in this context is evaluate and address the function/dysfunction of the ventral branch of the client's vagus nerve and the other four cranial nerves necessary for social engagement.

Many people who come to me have already been diagnosed by a medical doctor. I do treat people who have been given a medical diagnosis, primarily to improve the function of their nervous system. It has been my experience that bringing their autonomic nervous system into a state of social engagement and moving them toward optimal health has a positive effect and helps many of them with various medical issues.

In the initial interview, if clients tell me about a health issue, I make a note of it—can I relate their health issue to a possible dysfunction of one of the five cranial nerves involved in social engagement? I test the function of one branch of their vagus nerve. In some cases, I will test some of the other cranial nerves as well.

Then I have them do the Basic Exercise, or I administer one of the hands-on techniques described in Part Two, or other techniques from biomechanical craniosacral therapy. Then I test again. If we have brought about a positive change in the function of the ventral branch of the vagus nerve, there is a good chance that the client's body will self-regulate, and their health issues will be mitigated or even disappear.

My approach has helped many people with a wide range of problems including stress, psychological depression, migraines, fibromyalgia, difficulty in concentrating, remembering, or sleeping, problems with digestion, stiff neck, and back and shoulder pain.

We live in a world where everything is constantly changing, inside and outside of us. Our survival, wellness, and happiness depend on having a flexible autonomic nervous system that regulates us in order to respond appropriately to changes in our environment and our own organism.

CHAPTER 3

Neuroception and Faulty Neuroception

"Neuroception" is a term coined by Stephen Porges to describe how neural circuits distinguish whether a situation is safe, threatening, or dangerous. It is an ongoing process through which our autonomic nervous system evaluates information from our senses about our environment and the state of our body.

Neuroception takes place in the primitive parts of the brain, beyond our conscious awareness. It can be likened to a good watchdog that is always on guard, allowing us to focus on things other than survival, or to sleep soundly, and rousing us only when intrusions could compromise our survival. Based on the signals from neuroception, well-defined neural circuits are activated to support the state of social engagement and friendly communication behaviors when we are safe; the defensive strategies of fight or flight when we are threatened; and shutdown when we are in serious danger.[21]

Most people have their own experiences of neuroception when they accessed a "sixth sense" and knew that they were in danger or something was threatening, without consciously knowing how they knew it. A young woman in one of my classes once said, "I can have my back turned, and know that some guy I don't know is looking at me. I can feel his eyes on me before he comes up to me." Although we have no logical explanation for it, and even if we do not know its neural pathways, neuroception is far from uncommon.

Faulty Neuroception and Survival

Neuroception gives us access to information that we do not pick up with the conscious part of our mind. When it works properly, it is a true gift and can help us to survive. It works faster than processing conscious perceptions.

"I knew something was wrong even before I went into the room"—how do we pick up this kind of information? Sometimes we experience a conflict between our neuroception and other thoughts: "I had a feeling that something just wasn't right, but I allowed myself to be talked into going ahead with it anyway."

However, neuroception can be faulty, and when it does not work as it should we can find ourselves in deep trouble. Instead of clearly perceiving what is actually there, we distort what is going on. Faulty neuroception occurs when the neural circuits from perception to behavior do not function in an appropriate way. A person might react to a safe situation as if it were threatening or dangerous, or react to a dangerous situation as if it were safe.

There can be countless reasons for faulty neuroception. Our perception might be blinded by anger, fear, jealousy, or apathy, or we might be locked into a traumatic memory. We may be fixated in a state of shock; we may be hungry and have low blood sugar; we may be tired, in physical pain, or suffering from an illness.

We might be feeling perfectly normal and then suddenly be triggered by something that reminds us of a traumatic event in our past—and react to this memory as if it were happening in present time. We might not actually be threatened or endangered, but our nervous system may be stuck in the past, poised to fight or flee at the slightest trigger from the environment. A wonderful example of this is an Abbott and Costello sketch called "Slowly I Turned" (searchable on YouTube).

Faulty neuroception can even come from very positive experiences like falling in love and bonding with the partner. We sometimes hear that a person's judgment was impaired because they were "blinded by love," so that they failed to be aware of a possibly destructive situation.

The nervous system should be flexible, enabling our whole organism to adapt to the present situation and to support different kinds of behaviors depending on whether the situation is safe, threatening, or dangerous. In cases of chemical interference (such as prescription medicines, other drugs, and alcohol), information comes in from the environment through our senses, but the neural circuits do not process the information normally, and our physiology does not respond appropriately. Alcohol, for example, alters the way we feel and thus the way we act. Many drugs—prescription medicines as well as illegal and recreational drugs—also put us into an abnormal physiological and experiential state.

The following story illustrates faulty neuroception from biochemical interference. Three friends, young men in their mid-twenties, went for a daylong hike up Mount St. Helens, an active volcano in a national park in the southwest corner of the state of Washington. Although strenuous, this climb is suitable for anyone in good physical condition who is comfortable scrambling on steep, rugged terrain. Most climbers complete the round trip in seven to twelve hours.

The three friends prepared well for the hike; in each of their backpacks they had a map, compass, first-aid kit, and pocketknife with a set of tools. Each had good boots, a climbing helmet to protect his head from falling rocks, a lightweight sweater, sunscreen, and dust masks and goggles in the event of ash fall. The sun reflecting off snow and volcanic ash can be intense, so they also took sunglasses with side shields. They carried food and two quarts of water each.

They set off early in the morning. The weather forecast predicted a mild, sunny, clear day, and they dressed accordingly. They were soon quite warm from the sun and from their exertions, even though they were dressed only in T-shirts. They splashed water on their heads and took off their sweaty T-shirts.

The temperature of the body is regulated by neural feedback mechanisms that operate primarily through the hypothalamus, the part of the brain that processes information from key temperature sensors in the body. When the body starts to overheat, there are several physiological changes. When the temperature rises over 98.6° F (37° C), nerves to the blood vessels near the surface of the skin cause the blood vessels to dilate, increasing the amount of blood flowing to the skin. This is called vasodilation, and it enables more blood to reach the small capillaries in the skin. Up to a third of the body's blood can circulate in the skin, and is cooled at the skin surface by the surrounding air. Sweating also helps to cool the body as its moisture evaporates.

A few hours into the climb, the weather suddenly changed. Clouds formed, the air got cooler, and it began to snow. All three hikers felt cold, and they put on their sweaters. (They did not put their damp T-shirts back on.) Unfortunately, this layer of dry clothing did not provide sufficient warmth quickly enough, and they did not have rain gear. Within minutes, their sweaters were soaked from the cold, wet snow.

The hypothalamus works to conserve heat if the body temperature drops—autonomic heat-conserving responses are initiated as well as mechanisms that produce additional heat. A normal response to cold is the secretion of the stress hormones adrenaline (epinephrine), norepinephrine, and thyroxine. These cause the muscles to tighten, resulting in shivering. The activity from the rapid contractions of shivering muscles produces body heat.

Nerves during a stress response also cause contraction of the muscular walls of the blood vessels, called vasoconstriction. This minimizes heat loss by decreasing the volume of blood flowing from the core of the body to the skin, especially to the hands and feet.

One of the young climbers had taken his usual prescribed medication earlier in the day to suppress his chronic stress. One effect of this medicine is to lower blood levels of stress hormones. As a result, his body could not produce a normal stress reaction to cold weather. He did not shiver, his blood vessels did not constrict, his arteries and capillaries remained dilated, and the blood flow to his skin was not reduced to prevent further heat loss.

Because of the medicine, he was not able to adapt to the changes in his environment, and he became increasingly chilled. Cardiac arrest can occur in cases of extreme hypothermia, and finally his heart failed. This young hiker did not survive because his body was not able to adapt in normal ways to the weather shift.

This provides a cautionary tale about how chemical substances can interfere with our normal responses to dangerous situations, preventing our bodies from appropriately responding to protect us.

Other Causes of Faulty Neuroception

Earlier I described the survival value of the shutdown state. When a lion gets its jaws on the throat of an antelope or other prey, the autonomic nervous system of the prey usually goes into a state of shutdown in the face of imminent death and the inability to fight or flee anymore—and in some cases this can cause a predator to lose interest, which saves the life of its intended prey.

In contrast, personal problems in our complicated, modern, civilized human life are not usually so dramatic and usually last longer than a few seconds. We may not be threatened physically, but we are often challenged emotionally or mentally. We might need to get a project done on time, to address difficult issues in our relationships with the people around us, to solve an economic problem, or to care for a family member dying of cancer. We need to act—to do something or say something—in order to bring our world back to a state of temporary balance. We cannot always just sit on a beach, relax, and enjoy the surroundings.

Furthermore, unlike many wild animals, human beings do not usually shake off their traumas as soon as the threat or danger is gone. Ideally, we should be able to "reset" our nervous system and get a fresh start. But many times the effects of traumatic events stick with us long after the original shock. The conscious and unconscious memory can remain in our nervous system for months, years, or even for the rest of our lives. If we have not shaken it off, we can suffer from recurring inappropriate behaviors and ongoing physical symptoms of stress and shutdown.

Abnormal reactions to certain stimuli can occur because we once had a traumatic experience involving them. The psychological trigger causing a stress or shutdown reaction can be quite specific. The memory of the event sits like an unexploded land mine, waiting to be metaphorically stepped on by a soldier, or perhaps years later by an unsuspecting child. The reaction is triggered because something reminds us, consciously or unconsciously, of whatever traumatized us before.

The Story of Antaeus

The struggle between Antaeus and Heracles was a favorite subject in ancient and Renaissance sculpture.

Antaeus was the son of Poseidon, god of the sea, and Demeter, goddess of the Earth. The Greeks believed that he lived on the edge of the desert in what is now Libya. Antaeus would challenge all passersby to a wrestling match, kill them, and then use their skulls in a temple he was building to his father. Antaeus defeated all opponents until he fought Hercules.

Each time Hercules knocked him down, Antaeus got up and came back even stronger. Hercules quickly realized that he could not beat Antaeus by throwing him to the ground. He guessed the secret of Antaeus's power: when Antaeus came into contact with the Earth—his mother—he would be fortified and regain his strength.

Realizing this, Hercules grabbed Antaeus around the waist and held him aloft, breaking Antaeus's connection to the ground. Hercules was then able to use his colossal strength to crush him in a bear hug.

The story of Antaeus has been used to symbolize the dangers of not keeping ourselves grounded. Hercules displays the psychological and spiritual strength that accrues when, after being "upset," one becomes grounded again.

SENSING OUR OWN BODIES

Back in 1957, when I was sixteen and first learning how to play golf, I bought a book by Ben Hogan, one of the greatest early American professional golf champions. The book was *Ben Hogan's Five Lessons: The Modern Fundamentals of Golf.*[22] Hogan wrote, "If you want to hit a good drive, if you are right-handed, just keep your awareness on the little finger of your left hand as you swing the club."

Before I read that, I had tried to hit the ball as hard as I could, or to bring the club down as fast as I could. I did not understand what Ben Hogan wrote, but I tried it. And every time I remembered to sense that little finger, I got more distance when I hit the ball. Another result was that the ball went straight, toward the green almost every time. This was my first experience with the power of sensing my body.

Today there are many systems, including Pilates, yoga, martial arts, and mindfulness meditations, that help restore people to their sense of their body. If my clients have such a way of sensing their body, I ask them to use that. If not, I teach them an approach to help them do this.

The skin of the face is innervated by cranial nerve V, and the muscles of the face are innervated by CN VII. Light stroking of the face often calms us and helps us out of a state of stress. People very often unconsciously do this for themselves.

If I am giving them a massage, I can ask them to keep their attention on where my hands are touching their body. This is especially important for people in a state of withdrawal and dissociation—getting them back into a sense of their body becomes my first priority. I do not actually need to do anything. In that moment, when I have my hands on them, I am not trying to fix things or bring about any changes in their musculoskeletal structure. I am not relaxing a muscle, freeing the movement in a joint, adjusting the spine, or releasing connective tissue. Instead, my hands remain at the same place.

It is enough for me as the therapist to simply place my hands on the client's body, lightly touching the skin. Then I ask the client to "come to my hands with your awareness." At first, it can take some time for clients to clear their mind sufficiently of mental or emotional clutter in order to simply sense where their body is and what is going on in it. Therefore, I repeat the process several times. This is a simple way of helping clients to use their own sensing as a resource to get them grounded in their own body.

When I ask them to sense their body, I can take the same opportunity to sense my own body; I like to open my awareness to sense my own feet or hands, further grounding myself at the same time.

Sensing our own bodies and staying grounded helps us to remain in a ventral vagal state. Awareness of our body can help us avoid getting carried away by emotions that can lead to faulty neuroception.

CHAPTER 4

Testing the Ventral Branch of the Vagus Nerve

Simple Evaluation from Facial Observation

According to Stephen Porges, social engagement requires the ability to both look and listen. When you are talking with someone, you can sense whether or not he is socially engaged by how much he looks at you, how well he listens to you, and how well he can understand what you are saying. You can determine whether the person is looking and listening by reading the muscles of his face. Does the person look at your face and make eye contact with you, at least some of the time? Are his eyes open? Can he hear and understand what you are saying?

The muscles of the face are organized around the openings of the eyes, the nostrils, and the mouth. (See "Facial muscles" in the Appendix.) When these flat, round muscles tighten, they close the skin around the openings. Flat, rectangular muscles attach to the round muscles and can pull them more open, allowing more light to enter the eyes, more smells to enter the nose, and more air to enter the mouth. When we react emotionally, our facial expression changes as we open or close these openings.

Does the other person have slightly raised eyebrows, and are the eyes relaxed and open? The flat, round muscle that surrounds the eye is called the *orbicularis oculi*. (*Orbicularis* designates a muscle around a facial opening; *oculi* means related to the eyes.) By tightening this muscle, we close the opening around the eye, cutting down the amount of light in the same way that a shutter in an old reflex camera reduces the amount of light coming through the lens to the film.

We tighten this muscle to squint when we are exposed to bright light, when we wish to cut down on visual input, when there is something that we do not want to see emotionally, or when we want to withdraw from external sensory stimuli and contemplate our own thoughts. When we tighten this muscle, we move away from current visual stimuli, away from the here and now. We may remember events from the past, visualize future possibilities, or enter into a state of meditation.

When the flat, rectangular-shaped muscles above and below the *orbicularis oculi* are tense, they pull the *orbicularis oculi* more open, allowing much more light to come in. These muscles tense when we encounter something that is an "eye-opener." Physical tension in these flat rectangular muscles is an integral part of the emotional expression of surprise. It improves our sensory intake and helps us be more present to what is happening around us.

Strangely enough, when our eyes are more open, we can also hear better—there is a neurological connection between the nerves involved in sight and hearing. At a lecture, some people open their eyes slightly more in order to better hear what is being said.

When you make eye contact with another person, look for spontaneous facial expression in the middle third of her face (between the bottom of her eyes and the top of her mouth). The small movements here are an indication of social engagement (or lack of it) and the flexibility of her emotional responses.

There are two kinds of facial expression: those that we put on to show someone else what we feel, and those that occur without our consciously "making a face." We can categorize the latter into three types, depending on how long they last.

The first type of unconscious facial expression is the pattern of chronic tension, which is more or less permanent, etched into our faces with deep wrinkles and indicative of our characteristic emotional state.

The second pattern, of emotional tension, is less permanent and expresses our current mood. This pattern of facial tensions remains for a while—as long as a mood lasts, and generally long enough for someone else to get an impression of how we are feeling.

In the third kind of emotional expression, the facial muscles located in the band between the eyes and mouth change tension rapidly, up to several times a second. We can usually see these spontaneous micro-changes of expression in a baby or child. It is more rare to notice these changes in adults, as we are more locked into our sense of identity or moods. When these rapid changes are seen, they are too fast for us to read cognitively in order to say definitively that the facial expression indicates a certain emotion, but the fact that these spontaneous movements are there gives us a sense nonetheless that the person is open and without fear.

We can experience these rapid changes of facial expression when two people who feel safe with each other make eye contact, look at each other, and allow their feelings to flow without censoring or trying to control them. This is a reflection of the ideal state of openness, when our facial emotional expressions change as quickly as our thoughts. It is far different from a put-on smile, as when posing for a photo, where we almost grimace in an attempt to show positive feelings.

Can you see a flow of emotions on someone else's face—slight, rapidly changing, mercurial facial movements showing he feels happy, satisfied, angry, irritated, afraid, anxious, sad, or depressed—or is his face flat and unchanging, stuck in one emotional expression? Does he have melodic changes (prosody) in his vocal expression when he speaks? Or is his voice flat, with words spoken in a monotone?

We tend to think of people as unchanging identities. However, their interactions with other people are affected by their mood, which is affected by the state of their autonomic nervous system at that moment.

People in a stress state might look at us in a menacing way, and their attitude might be aggressive. They might not listen to what is being said. They can be prone to react to a single word, to fly off the handle and interrupt us in the middle of a sentence. Often we may need to correct them: "But that is not what I said!"

People in fear will avoid eye contact with us, or make eye contact for only a split second and then look away. Their breathing might be shallow, lifting only the ribs of their upper chest, and they might hold their breath after the inbreath.

People in a depressed state will tip their heads forward or let their heads hang, with an expressionless face. They move slowly, indicating a lack of energy. They have no enthusiasm, and do not want to engage in conversation. Sometimes, before a depressed person does or says something, she will breathe out or sigh.

OTHER TESTS OF VAGAL FUNCTION

In my clinic, in addition to observing aspects such as these, I like to start all my treatments by testing for function of the ventral vagus nerve branch. If a client exhibits some of the symptoms that I describe as the "heads of the Hydra" (see list at the beginning of Part One), and if testing her indicates ventral vagal dysfunction, it's often possible to improve the person's condition by using the exercises and techniques described in Part Two.

Then, after the client does the Basic Exercise, or after I treat her with my hands, I test again for ventral vagal function to be sure that we have achieved the desired results. This information is useful in a clinical setting; the procedure described below in a later section of this chapter, which makes it possible to evaluate our own ventral vagal function, is also useful for self-diagnosis and self-care as well as helping others.

In addition to looking at the back of the throat and having the person say "ah-ah-ah," as I describe later, I sometimes use another test that is useful if I am testing a young child, an autistic individual, or others in extenuating circumstances. For example, if I have a class of second graders, it might start them all laughing if they see me looking into a classmate's throat with a little flashlight and asking her to say "ah-ah-ah."

This other test is based on the observation by Mayer, Traube, and Hering in the late nineteenth century that the pulse and blood pressure should be faster and stronger on the inbreath than on the outbreath (assuming good function of the ventral vagus nerve). As you gain experience treating many people, you can get a sense that one person has a greater difference than someone else. You might also observe that the difference is greater after she has done the Basic Exercise than it was before.

It is my experience that people who have a greater difference between the pulses during their inbreaths and outbreaths are usually more robust and healthy, both physically and psychologically.

However, these tests that I use in my clinic have limitations for purposes of scientific research. They are subjectively based on my personal observations, which only show whether or not the ventral branch of the vagus nerve is functional; they do not quantify the level of vagal function, which can be higher in one person than in another. Other options for testing for vagal function are described below.

Objectively Evaluating Vagal Function through Heart Rate Variability (HRV)

In scientific research on the autonomic nervous system, there is increasing awareness of *heart rate variability,* which may offer us another way to assess vagal nerve function.

When our nervous system is functioning optimally and we are socially engaged, there are differences in the length of time between consecutive heartbeats, resulting from the natural rise and fall of the heart rate in response to breathing, blood pressure, hormones, and emotions. Heart rate variability (HRV) is the measurement of these differences. Greater variation in the time intervals is designated as high HRV.

HRV can be used as an indicator of general health.[23] It represents one of the most promising evaluative tools to measure autonomic nervous system activity.[24] When the ventral branch of the vagus nerve functions properly, heart rate variability is high. There is a growing amount of research correlating high HRV with health and longevity.[25]

On the other hand, when there is a reduced level of function in the ventral vagus, the person's autonomic nervous system reverts to either a stress state or a state of dorsal vagal activity, as described in the previous chapter. In this case, differences in the time intervals between heartbeats are smaller or nonexistent, and this is designated as low HRV.

A growing body of scientific studies shows a correlation between low heart rate variability and various psychological/psychiatric problems.

For example, HRV is related to emotional states, and has been found to decrease under conditions of acute time pressure, post-traumatic stress, emotional strain, and elevated state anxiety.[26] Individuals reporting a greater frequency and duration of daily worry are found to have a lower HRV.[27,28]

Low HRV is apparently also related to a lack of ability to concentrate, and to motor inhibition, both of which are symptoms commonly found in children with ADHD.[29] There is also a link between post-traumatic stress disorder and low heart rate variability.[30]

In terms of physical health, it is hypothesized that low HRV is an indicator of less favorable health in general.[31] A range of adverse health conditions may be associated with lower HRV: obesity, diabetic neuropathy, activity of the dorsal branch of the vagus nerve, susceptibility to sudden infant death syndrome (SIDS), and poor survival rates in premature babies.

People suffering from obesity generally have lower HRV.[32] While we might assume that overweight people eat too much, exercise too little, and lack the motivation to change their behavior, some overweight people go on a diet and almost starve themselves with little improvement in their weight. Some people wanting to lose weight work with a psychologist or hypnotherapist to change their self-image. I cannot help but speculate: what if their program for weight loss included evaluation of their HRV, and improvement of their social engagement nervous system with the Basic Exercise?

Many people with sexual dysfunction seek help from their medical doctor or advice from a psychiatrist or psychologist. A recent study sheds some light on women's sexual dysfunction, indicating that it may be closely linked to their heart rate variability.[33] There are studies that draw a similar conclusion regarding erectile dysfunction in men, noting that "general imbalance of the autonomic nervous system is one of the causes of erectile dysfunction."[34]

Studies of HRV have shown that low HRV was found in people with heart damage,[35] and it has been associated with increased risk of coronary heart disease.[36] Reduced HRV also appears to be a predictor of mortality after myocardial infarction (heart attack).[37]

Low HRV correlates with early death from several causes in addition to heart problems, such as COPD. In the United States in 2014, COPD was the third most common cause of death after heart disease and cancer.[38] Breathing patterns other than normal diaphragmatic breathing indicate lower levels of physical and psychological health, and there is a relationship between diaphragmatic breathing and higher levels of heart rate variability.[39] In my clinic, I have found that clients with a diagnosis of COPD have very little movement in their respiratory diaphragm, and their tests do not show ventral vagal activity.

HRV testing, it seems, may yield valuable diagnostic information, and can serve as a rapid screening tool to evaluate altered autonomic nervous system activity.

If scientific research confirms that the state of the autonomic nervous system is a factor in psychological issues, it may be interesting to explore the possibility of improving heart rate variability and the function of the ventral branch of the vagus nerve as a first step in treating psychological problems, without immediately resorting to traditional psychological interventions or prescription drugs. (See Chapter 6 for more on this topic.)

Testing for Vagal Function: Early Experiences

Let me emphasize the importance of testing by recollecting my practice in earlier days. When I started my education in craniosacral therapy, the teacher of the course said that if I did the fixed sequence of techniques that he taught, I could help people to get relief from their stress. However, he never taught us to test the physiological states of the body, so I wondered how he knew that these techniques worked—perhaps he had simply heard that from his teacher, and believed it.

That was almost thirty years ago, before I studied with Alain Gehin, and long before I heard about the Polyvagal Theory. The only model of stress we had at that time was the old understanding of the autonomic nervous system being in a state of either stress or relaxation.

Everyone knew that chronic stress was unhealthy, and there were books and courses on stress management, each promising a positive, stress-free outcome. But none of them showed a way of testing stress physiologically. Today I test every patient before and after sessions; I do not put my blind faith in what someone else once told me about what outcome to expect from my treatments.

When I did sessions based on that first course, I completed the standard sequence of techniques, and assumed that my work was finished; the client could no longer be stressed, and was relaxed and ready to go home. But I noticed that clients often had a hard time gathering themselves after treatment, and they would ask if they could remain on the table for a few more minutes. After ten or fifteen minutes, they often still did not want to get up, and I would have to explain that I needed the massage table for my next client. They would be considerate of my needs, get up reluctantly, and put their shoes on. I remember some clients asking me if I thought that they could drive; I assured them that it was okay.

When they came for their next appointment, they sometimes told me that they were so relaxed after their last session that they had to pull off to the side of the road and shut their eyes to nap for a few minutes. Sometimes they even pulled over two or three times. They enthusiastically commented that this was great because they had been "so relaxed." Even on the next day, they often did not want to get out of bed and go to work.

Today, looking back, I realize that my sessions had left them in a dorsal vagal state. They were not relaxed, but instead were dissociated and exhibiting depressive behavior. Nowadays, I am careful to address ventral vagal function during a session, and test it again afterward, in order to make sure that they can be socially engaged when they depart. I make sure that they leave my office calm but at the same time alert and able to function, in a state of neither stress nor dorsal vagal activity. Testing the state of the autonomic nervous system before and after a session provides a great perspective if you are a body therapist, psychologist, or any other kind of health care provider.

Discovering the Polyvagal Theory

In the early 1980s, I began to notice that many of my clinical clients who had asthma also had vagal dysfunction. When I helped them to improve their vagal function, their symptoms of asthma were reduced or disappeared.

I found this interesting—perhaps people with asthma could be helped by hands-on treatment to improve their ventral vagal function rather than relying on prescription medications, which are expensive and often have negative side effects. I hope someday to do a scientific study based on these experiences.

At the time, I used a method of testing vagal function that was based on early concepts of heart rate variability: I monitored the pulse and blood pressure of my clients, and correlated these with their breathing. I learned this method from my Rolfing teachers, Michael Salveson and Gael Ohlgren, in 1982–83. My teachers had learned it from Peter Levine,[40] a leading teacher and author in the field of trauma therapy. Peter in turn had been inspired by Stephen Porges; Peter and Stephen have a friendship that goes back several decades. Michael and Peter were also part of a small study group of Rolfers and other body therapists in Berkeley, California, in the early 1980s that focused on the function of the autonomic nervous system.

The method I used involved observation of the breath and pulse. If our pulse is faster on the inbreath and slower on the outbreath, this indicates good ventral vagal function. The greater the difference, the better the ventral vagal function. I monitored this by putting a finger over an artery in the client's wrist while at the same time observing the pattern of her breathing. The idea behind this method goes back to studies on the autonomic nervous system from the 1890s, with the discovery of variability in blood pressure described as Traube-Hering-Mayer waves.

Although this method was useful in my clinic for my own personal evaluation, it left a lot to be desired in terms of scientific research. I had no objective measurement of vagal function—just my subjective impression based on what I felt under my fingers and saw with my eyes. For scientific purposes, of course, it is preferable to measure more precisely. Today there are many instruments available to measure vagal function.[41]

Back in 2002, I wanted to ask Stephen Porges (whom I had not yet met) to help me develop a research project investigating my successful hands-on treatment for asthma. Several clients had come to me with breathing difficulties and diagnoses of asthma. When I tested these clients before their first session (using a method of diagnosing the function of the vagus nerve that I had learned in my Rolfing class), I noticed that they all had vagal dysfunction. But after my hands-on treatments, they all tested positive for vagal function. At the same time, their symptoms of asthma disappeared, and their breathing normalized. I was hoping that Stephen could assist me in developing a scientifically acceptable method of measuring this.

I asked Jim Oschman,[42] a scientist friend of mine, if he knew Stephen and could introduce me to him. Luckily, on my next trip to the United States to visit my family in Philadelphia, Stephen Porges was giving a lecture in Baltimore for the American Association of Body Psychotherapists. Jim was in Washington, DC, and all three of us were able to meet at the Baltimore conference and have dinner together.

I told Stephen about my idea for doing a research project on treating asthma, and I asked if he could help me measure autonomic nervous system function before and after my treatments. Rather than supplying information on where I could get the hardware and software, as I had hoped, he changed the subject and told us about his Polyvagal Theory. It was new to me, but it sounded interesting. The next morning, Jim and I had breakfast with Stephen, and he told us more about the theory.

Later that morning, Stephen gave the keynote speech at the conference. His theme was the Polyvagal Theory, this time illustrated with slides. After hearing Stephen describe the theory for the third time in less than twenty-four hours, I began to truly grasp it.

He presented video documentaries showing some of the improvements in communication and behavior in autistic children who had taken part in his research, which he calls "The Listening Project Protocol"[43] (further described in Chapter 7). The children had received five daily forty-five-minute treatments for five days, consisting of listening to unique computer-distorted music through special headphones. The result was that more than half of the subjects no longer reported auditory hyperacusis, and many started to engage spontaneously in two-way verbal communication, and became more social.

The video showed the children's interaction with an adult who tried to engage them in playful activity that fit their age group—the therapist was blowing soap bubbles. Before the music-listening sessions, one child was hyperactive, could not sit still, ran around in circles, and showed no interest in either the adult or the bubbles. Another child was sitting passively, with her chin drooping on her chest. By contrast, she seemed to be collapsed, alone in her own world, and did not appear to notice the bubbles or the adult.

After their fifth listening sessions, both children looked engaged and behaved more naturally. The formerly hyperactive child stood in front of the adult, made eye contact, and played with the soap bubbles. The child who had been shut down appeared to wake from her stupor, related playfully to the adult, and started to play with the soap bubbles as well. The children smiled, laughed, had light in their eyes, and were in a playful, relaxed, and open state.

This is an incredible accomplishment, given the fact that until then no one had developed a scientifically verified procedure for helping autistic people improve their communication skills and become more social. The Listening Project Protocol points to a potential for effectively addressing this symptom of autism.

I was not the only one who was amazed. The room was filled with 150 therapists. After seeing the impact of this intervention on the two children, there was not a dry eye in the house.

At that time, I had no experience treating children on the autism spectrum. I thought about patients I had treated over the years. Many had come to my clinic in a state of stress or dorsal vagal withdrawal, and had left smiling, with light in their eyes and apparently at peace with themselves. This indicated to me that our sessions had been effective.

I believed that I had the means to bring about similar changes in autistic clients with a protocol of techniques from biomechanical craniosacral therapy. However, before hearing Stephen Porges's lecture, I did not have a psycho-physiological model to explain the changes. Also, I realized that my previous model of the autonomic nervous system was limited to states of either stress or relaxation. My model did not include the idea of "shutdown," or any state characterized by activity of the dorsal vagal branch; it did not even distinguish between the ventral and dorsal branches of the vagus nerve.

I came away from Stephen's lecture inspired, and my interest shifted from doing research on treating asthma with craniosacral therapy to exploring the possibility of treating children on the autism spectrum.

I also had a new understanding of how the autonomic nervous system functions. It was no longer a question of improving just vagal function, but improving the function of the four other cranial nerves also essential for social engagement. I have spent the many years since then studying and applying the Polyvagal Theory in my clinical practice and in my teaching.

When I went home to Denmark, I could not set up a lab to do the kind of testing that Porges had done, and I did not have access to his process of testing and acoustic stimulation. But I decided to work with certain clients on the autism spectrum using my new knowledge of the Polyvagal Theory and my hands-on skills from biomechanical craniosacral therapy, which include techniques for improving the function of the five cranial nerves necessary for social engagement.

My hope was that, by using those techniques and improving the function of those nerves, I could also help some of these people improve their ability to communicate, thus making it possible for them to engage more fully in social behavior.

My treatments resulted in better functioning for most of my autistic clients. They did become more communicative and went from states of isolation to becoming more socially responsive. Although I used a different therapeutic approach from that of Stephen Porges, I based my treatments on his Polyvagal Theory.

It took several years to reach a point where I realized the importance of testing everyone, even after hearing about the Polyvagal Theory. At first I measured vagal function only when I had a difficult patient and felt frustrated with a lack of results; I was slow to incorporate it for all my clients.

When I gave a myofascial release treatment but did not get the result I expected, I would hit a wall—these techniques usually worked, so why not this time? So I worked harder, repeating the same technique again and again, and giving my clients extra time for their sessions. Even with that, my efforts still did not give the results that I wanted, and I became more and more frustrated and unsatisfied at the end of a session.

Testing for vagal function gave me a chance to realize that my failures were not due to my lack of judgment in choosing that technique, or skill at performing it, but rather to a lack of receptivity in the client's nervous system. In these cases, information about the state of their autonomic nervous system helped me understand why I did not get the results I had attained with most of my other clients who had well-functioning autonomic nervous systems.

With this realization, I no longer questioned my ability as a therapist when I had a difficult case; the shortcoming was not in me or my technique, but was due to the unreceptive state of the client's autonomic nervous system. What would happen if I had the information about their autonomic nervous system issues at the start of the session, and addressed that first? I began to do this.

Based on my resultant clinical successes, I believe that the importance of testing for the function of the ventral branch of the vagus nerve cannot be overestimated. Whether my clients come for a Rolfing session, to get relief from pain in their back, or to regain mobility in a frozen shoulder—or for any other of the health issues that I call the "heads of the Hydra"—the first thing that I do is test them for function of the ventral branch of their vagus nerve, using the pharyngeal-branch vagal function test described below, since my first goal as a therapist is to improve their vagal function.

If I find ventral vagal dysfunction, indicating a state of either stress or withdrawal, I have the client do the Basic Exercise (see Part Two). Then

I test them again. Usually their vagus nerve responds as it should after doing this exercise once or twice. Then I proceed with specific techniques to complete the treatment.

I have learned that if there is not adequate ventral vagal function, therapeutic interventions are less likely to stick. However, when vagal function is successfully restored, my clients often experience improvements in other areas of their lives—not only in terms of the health issue that they came in with, but also at work, with their families, and in social relationships with others.

Testing another person for social engagement can be valuable if you are working as a teacher, body therapist, psychologist, psychiatrist, or coach. If you are a parent about to send a child to college, it might be a good idea to make sure that your child has a well-functioning autonomic nervous system—and if not, it would be a good idea to get it functional, to ensure the best chance that the time and resources you and your child invest in the education will have a positive outcome. If you find that your child is in a state of stress or withdrawal, you might want to address that with the exercises and treatments in this book, for the best possible chance of success.

Testing for Vagal Function: Cottingham, Porges, and Lyon

If you are a body therapist, or do anything else to help other people with their health and wellness, performance, or interactions with others, you might find that the state of their autonomic nervous system will predict how successful your efforts will be.

Stephen Porges, together with John Cottingham and Todd Lyon, both Rolfers, published the results of a 1988 research project in the journal *Physical Therapy*.[44] They demonstrated that evaluation of the autonomic nervous system can be an accurate predictor of the level of success in a hands-on therapy session. Over the years, I have found that the implications of this study go far beyond body therapy, and are relevant in all interactions.

The three did a scientific experiment on a group of men in which they tested the state of the autonomic nervous system and how it related to the level of positive results from a myofascial release technique used in Rolfing.

John Cottingham administered a Rolfing technique called a "pelvic lift" to each of the study participants. The pelvic lift is used to balance the sacrum at the end of Rolfing sessions, in order to incorporate and balance changes to the connective tissue from various releases that occurred during the session.

In the pelvic lift technique, the client lies face-up on a massage table. The Rolfer slides a hand under the client's sacrum and contacts the bone. With the client's weight resting on the palm of their hand, the Rolfer creates a slight, steady, gentle traction toward the client's feet. When the pelvic lift works as intended, the muscles of the back relax, the spine lengthens, and vertebral alignment is improved. The pelvic lift should leave the client with better posture, greater flexibility in the lumbar spine, and an increased sense of well-being.

For the purposes of the study, in order to keep the intervention as uniform as possible for all of the subjects, John Cottingham was the only therapist, administering the same technique to all the subjects.

John measured the effects of his technique by testing the flexibility of the spine before and after the pelvic lift. The subjects started in a relaxed standing posture, and then curled forward into spinal flexion. John measured how close their fingertips came to touching the floor, both before and afterward, to determine whether the subject was more flexible, the same, or less flexible after the pelvic lift. John asked them how they felt, and what they experienced as a result of receiving the pelvic lift. Even with the same therapist doing the same technique, there was a wide range of responses.

From a first glance at the findings, it appeared that the younger men generally had a more positive gain from the technique compared with the older men, showing an increased range of movement when they bent over the second time. They reported that receiving a pelvic lift had been an enjoyable experience, and they were in a better mood after the intervention.

The older group had quite different results. In spite of John's training, skills, and positive intention, his efforts with many of the older men were not especially successful. Many became stiffer and actually lost some of their range of movement; when they curled forward and tried to touch their toes, their fingers were further from the floor than before the treatment. Many reported that they did not feel as good after the technique, and their mood had changed for the worse. A few were noticeably grumpier and more irritable.

It would be easy to conclude that Rolfing simply works better for younger men than for older men. But the researchers were interested in relating the results of the technique to a factor other than age. They discovered that the state of the autonomic nervous system was a relevant indicator in predicting the success of the outcome.

Before the treatments in the experiment, John measured the subjects' heart rate variability (HRV). He attached sensors to their skin and ran these wires to a vagal-tone monitor stationed in another room. With this setup, he was able to precisely record changes in the beating of their hearts, and to correlate them to individual breaths.

John was not able to see the HRV measurements while carrying out the technique. He had no knowledge of which subjects had high levels of heart rate variability and which had low levels, so this knowledge could not prejudice the way that he performed the treatments. Most of the younger subjects, and some of the older men, had reasonably high heart rate variability. By contrast, a higher percentage of the older men and only a few of the younger men had low HRV.

When Cottingham, Porges, and Lyon reviewed the data, they saw a closer relationship between high heart rate variability and a desirable outcome from the treatment than there was between age and outcome. In other words, the success of the treatment appeared to be more closely related to the state of the autonomic nervous system than to age. This is a key point, discussed further below.

Measuring heart rate variability with a vagal tone monitor can be useful in scientific research where you need a quantifiable measurement.

However, there are other ways to evaluate vagal function in a clinical setting that do not require special equipment and take less time. For many years, I have used some of these other methods and found them to be sufficient for my own purposes in my clinic.

A Simple Test of the Pharyngeal Vagus Branch

The ventral vagus nerve has several branches. Below is a test for the func-tion of one of these, called the pharyngeal branch, which inner-vates the part of the throat immediately behind the nasal cavity and the mouth, above the esophagus and larynx. Nerve fibers from the pharyngeal branch of the vagus go to the soft palate and to the pharynx. This nerve is involved with swallowing and making vocal sounds.

The Greek physician Claudius Galen was the first extant writer to describe the pharyngeal branch of the vagus nerve, noting that it provided motor nerve function for the muscles in the larynx, which produce the voice. He learned this by examining a gladiator who had been wounded in the neck and had lost his voice; Galen found that the pharyngeal branch of his vagus nerve had been severed on one side of his neck. To test the validity of his observations, he did an experiment on pigs, whose anatomy is quite similar to human beings. He found that cutting the pharyngeal nerve on pigs would stop their squealing.

After trying various ways of testing the ventral branch of the vagus nerve, I eventually chose this method focusing on its pharyngeal branch. It has been described in some of the older textbooks on anatomy and physiology, and it is still taught in medical schools in Denmark. Alain Gehin also taught this method of testing for vagus function by looking at the back of the throat. It has been a great asset in terms of my own work with craniosacral therapy.

This test evaluates the movement of one of the muscles innervated by the pharyngeal branch, called the *levator veli palatini* muscle. From my experience, I find that the condition of this branch is a good indicator of the function of other branches of the ventral vagus nerve as well.

Improving the function of the pharyngeal branch of the vagus nerve improves the function of the respiratory diaphragm. When this test shows a dysfunction of the *levator veli palatini* muscle, I usually also observe that the client's breathing is irregular, somewhat rapid, and not especially deep. Then, after the client does the Basic Exercise and this branch becomes functional again, I observe that breathing has improved, becoming deeper and slower.

I explain to my clients the importance of proper function in the ventral branch of their vagus nerve. I show them drawings, and I explain what I am looking for in terms of movement of their soft palate at the back of their throat. Most of my clients like the idea that I test vagal function, treat them, and then test vagal function again; they like the fact that their autonomic nervous system can be evaluated, and if the ventral branch of their vagus nerve has been dysfunctional, that it can be shown to be brought back into proper function.

How to Test for Pharyngeal Ventral Branch Function

Ask the person to sit comfortably in a chair. Then stand in front of him and ask him to open his mouth so that you can see the back of his throat. You will need to see the uvula (the small bulb-shaped structure that hangs down in the back of the throat) and the soft-tissue arches on either side of it. Sometimes you can see these sufficiently with normal light; otherwise, you will need to use a small flashlight. (The flashlight app on an iPhone is perfect for this.)

If the person's tongue is blocking your view of the uvula and arches, ask him to place one of his fingers on the back of his tongue and push it down onto the floor of his mouth. Then you should be able to see the soft palate more easily. (Medical doctors use a tongue depressor for this, but that makes some people gag, and I have never had a client gag using his own finger.)

See the Appendix for a series of drawings of the uvula. In "Uvula 2," the arches of the soft palate are lifted on both sides by properly functioning *levator veli palatini* muscles. In "Uvula 3," one side is lifted and the other is not; this indicates dysfunction of the ventral branch of the vagus nerve on the side that is not lifted.

In these drawings, you can see the *levator veli palatini* muscles embedded in the soft tissue, one on either side of the uvula. These muscles are innervated by motor fibers of the pharyngeal branch of the vagus nerve. When they contract, they lift the arches of the soft palate. They are also attached to the auditory (Eustachian) tube between the ears and throat, and pull on it during the act of swallowing. This is why the ears sometimes "pop" with swallowing, as air moves into the middle-ear cavity and pressure is equalized.

When we swallow, these muscles should contract, elevating the soft palate and allowing food to go into the esophagus en route to the stomach, while at the same time preventing food from entering the larynx and lungs. These muscles should also contract when someone makes the sound "ah." A well-trained singer will use this muscle to lift the back of the throat before singing the first note of a phrase.

In order to test vagal function, I ask the other person to say, "ah-ah-ah-ah-ah" while I observe the arches on either side of the uvula. These sounds should be percussive and staccato—short, distinct bursts of sound in quick succession, and not a long, drawn-out "aaaaaaaaahhhh," which does not create the desired effect. If there is good function in the pharyngeal branch of the ventral vagus nerve on both the right and left sides, these muscles tighten symmetrically with a clear impulse when the person makes the sounds "ah-ah-ah-ah-ah," lifting the arches of the soft palate equally on both sides.

If, on the other hand, there is dysfunction of the pharyngeal branch of the ventral branch of the vagus nerve on one side, the nerve impulses do not innervate the *levator veli palatini* muscle on that side, and the arch in the soft palate on that side does not lift when the person says "ah."

This test for ventral vagal function has profound implications. As mentioned, if we are in a state of fear, there is activity in one of these other two circuits of the autonomic nervous system, and we can suffer from any of the conditions I referred to as the "heads of the Hydra." Stephen

Porges introduced the idea of the "vagal brake"—the inhibitory effect of ventral vagus activity on spinal sympathetic and dorsal vagal activity.

What if we then came to feel safe? What if we restored activity in our ventral vagal circuit instead of our spinal sympathetic chain or dorsal vagal branch?

The exercises and treatments in this book can move someone out of states of stress or shutdown and into a ventral vagal state. After someone does the self-help exercises or receives the hands-on treatments in this book, you should be able to observe improvement when you test again—the soft palate and the uvula should now lift symmetrically on both sides.

The "Trap Squeeze Test" is another test that I use to test for the function of the ventral vagus nerve branch. This test and its implications are described in Chapter 5. It is perfect to use with children, or with anyone on the autistic spectrum who might have difficulty following your instructions.

Therapists Can Test for Vagal Function without Touching

In January 2008, I co-taught a seminar together with Stephen Porges in Santa Fe, New Mexico, for a large group of psychologists and body therapists. Stephen began the seminar, and everyone was inspired by his presentation of the Polyvagal Theory, recognizing its possibilities as a model for understanding the difference between normal and abnormal human behavior.

Psychologists interact verbally with their clients and are regulated by laws governing their professional behavior. In most states in the United States, they are not allowed to touch their clients; doing so would be grounds for losing their license. My work with clients, however, is primarily "hands-on," for body therapists who want to learn how to use their hands to treat their client in this way.

The night before I lectured to this group, I wondered, "These psychologists cannot touch their clients. How can I give them something that they can take home and use in their clinical practice?" I slept on the question, and the next morning, when I woke up, I had an answer: they could diagnose the state of the client's autonomic nervous system by looking at the back of the throat while the client makes the sound "ah-ah-ah-ah-ah" (as described in the section above).

I provided each of the seminar participants with a small flashlight to enable them to look at the back of someone's throat. In a practice session during the course, they experimented with testing other seminar attendees. The point was for them to learn how to tell whether or not their clients were socially engaged, both before and after their verbal interventions—such testing might help them to better understand the behavior and emotional state of their client from a Polyvagal perspective. They could also evaluate whether their clients needed work to improve the function of their autonomic nervous system and, just as importantly, whether their intervention was successful in terms of the Polyvagal Theory. The possibility of testing before and after a session caught their interest.

I told them about my work with body therapy, and the research done by Porges, Cottingham, and Lyon described above. I raised the possibility of a psychologist having clients use their own hands to perform a technique that could facilitate a change in their autonomic nervous system, bringing them from a state of chronic spinal sympathetic or dorsal vagal activity into a state of social engagement.

If Stephen Porges's vagal brake can be brought into play—if a psychologist can get a client's ventral vagal branch to function properly, "putting the brake on" sympathetic or dorsal vagal activity and their harmful consequences—what effects might this have on the behavior, emotions, and thoughts of the client? Since the ventral branch of the vagus nerve inhibits dorsal vagal or spinal sympathetic activity, bringing about a ventral vagal state may be effective in addressing conditions often diagnosed as stress or depression.

Although in my clinic I utilized a hands-on protocol to bring my clients into a state of social engagement, I reasoned that a psychologist who understood the Polyvagal Theory could use its principles to teach clients to achieve similar results using their own hands. Such an approach would also give clients the possibility of helping themselves in the future, after the session, to regulate their own autonomic nervous system as needed.

This was the origin of the Basic Exercise. (See Part Two for instructions for doing this simple exercise.)

This was the first time that I had taught this exercise to anyone, and naturally I was curious whether or not it would work. There were about sixty psychologists in the group, and half of them had shown vagal dysfunction when tested prior to doing the exercise. (Their partners in the practice session never touched them.) After they used their own hands to treat themselves, they all showed restored ventral vagal function. Bringing about the change in their autonomic nervous systems had taken only a few minutes.

After the seminar, I received an email from one of the psychologists, telling me that she now tested every client at the start of their sessions. If they had vagal dysfunction, she told them how to do the exercise. When she tested them again afterward, they showed ventral vagus function. This exercise, it appeared, successfully put her patients into a state of social engagement. Then she did her usual verbal psychological interventions. She wrote that she was thrilled by the improved results that she was now getting with her clients.

When I went back to work in my own clinic, I began asking whether patients had physical or psychological problems. I checked them to see if they had ventral vagal function. Then I taught them to do the Basic Exercise. When they had done it a single time, I looked at the back of their throat again, and each and every one of them now had a well-functioning ventral vagus nerve.

I would have been satisfied if I had helped 50 percent of my patients to a ventral vagal state, but I found that I was able to help them all. Eighty-five out of the next eighty-five clients I tracked had a positive outcome. That was a good enough result for me to begin to depend on this exercise. Clients, furthermore, usually gave me good feedback not only at the end of the session but also when I saw them again in the following weeks.

CHAPTER 5

The Polyvagal Theory— A New Paradigm for Health Care?

Generally, our Western approach to medical treatment is biochemical or surgical. If we go to a doctor with a health problem, the doctor listens to our description of the problem. After a physical examination and/ or laboratory testing, the doctor generally makes a diagnosis, writes a prescription for medication, and sometimes suggests a surgical procedure.

If we have asthma, doctors prescribe asthma medicine. If we have migraines, they prescribe migraine medicine. If we are having a problem with digestion, they prescribe a specific medicine to help a specific part of the digestive tract. There is a different medicine for every nameable condition; a well-stocked pharmacy offers thousands of medicines.

In the conventional approach, however, doctors may be overlooking something. Dysfunction of the autonomic nervous system, for instance, may be a common factor in autism, migraines, COPD, and many other health problems.

Rather than focusing on one diagnosis or condition that is treated by one medicine, there is a growing awareness of comorbidity. Comorbidity is the presence of one or more disorders or diseases co-occurring with a primary disease or disorder. The additional disorder(s) might be behavioral or psychological.

The autonomic nervous system monitors and regulates the functioning of the visceral organs, and is a major contributing factor in determining our emotional state. However, doctors do not usually test its function; they do not generally consider the autonomic nervous system as a possible contributing factor, nor are they trained to explore the possibility of changing the state of the autonomic nervous system without using prescription medicines.

In my practice, I have consistently found that assisting the ventral branch of the vagus nerve to function properly often eliminates or reduces the severity of many health problems, and therefore the need for prescription drugs.

I believe dysfunction of those nerves to be an underlying cause of many life-impairing physiological and behavioral conditions. I invite you to explore this approach in greater depth after reading this book. Whether you are a layperson, health care professional, or body therapist, I trust that you will find the concepts and techniques as effective as I have found them in my own practice.

A Polyvagal Approach for Psychological and Physical Conditions

Many people focus on the negative consequences of stress and are generally not aware of problems resulting from chronic activation of the dorsal branch of the vagus nerve. Activity of the dorsal vagus is characterized by a lack of physical energy, low blood pressure, fainting, breathing difficulties stemming from constriction of the airways in cases of COPD, and chronic, general muscle and joint pain, often diagnosed as fibromyalgia.[45,46]

As described in Chapter Two, chronic dorsal vagal activity is also a factor in depressive behavior, social isolation, feelings of helplessness and hopelessness, apathy, lack of empathy, sadness, and grief, as well as some cases of post-traumatic stress and many cases of anxiety.

Prior to the Polyvagal Theory, we did not have an adequate physiological model to understand the nature of these common problems. The new understanding of the autonomic nervous system set forth in the Polyvagal Theory provides us with a physiological model for comprehending the neurological factors underlying these dysfunctions. Improving the function of the ventral branch of the vagus nerve opens new possibilities for healing a myriad of health problems arising from chronic sympathetic-system activation or dorsal-vagal dysfunction.

Stephen Porges elucidated how our autonomic nervous system affects us mentally, physically, and emotionally. He postulated that physiological factors such as the autonomic nervous system and hormonal levels play a role in determining our psychological state and therefore our behavior. If we want to change our psychological state and behavior patterns, or help others change theirs, the solutions might lie in initiating changes in the state of the autonomic nervous system.

The implications of Stephen Porges's theory carry the potential to develop and implement many new treatments. Perhaps we will not have to rely as much on antidepressants or other mood enhancers, which are expensive, often do not work as desired, and in some cases have serious negative side effects.[47]

BUILDING ON STEPHEN PORGES'S SUCCESS

For fifteen years before I met Stephen Porges, I had been working with biomechanical craniosacral therapy, a form of hands-on manipulation to improve the function of the cranial nerves.[48] The biomechanical approach to craniosacral therapy includes tests for the function of the cranial nerves as well as techniques to remove restrictions in the sutures (bone junctions) of the cranium in order to improve the function of the cranial nerves.

After meeting Stephen in 2002, I developed a craniosacral therapy protocol by choosing several of Alain Gehin's techniques. Together these techniques usually establish proper function of the ventral branch of the vagus and the other four cranial nerves necessary for social engagement. I have taught this protocol to more than five hundred craniosacral therapists in Denmark and Norway, and it has proven to be successful in regulating their clients' autonomic nervous systems. In many cases, the positive results have been astounding, and there are no negative side effects.

I would like nothing more than to be able to pass on this knowledge to all therapists who are interested. However, these techniques are usually communicated in a direct transmission between a teacher and students in small classes. It takes a long time for students to learn and to master the techniques.

My first thought when I started to write this book was to introduce the Polyvagal Theory and then present a description of how to do these techniques. However, there are major challenges in teaching these advanced techniques through a book, especially to people with no prior skills or knowledge of the craniosacral system.

So instead I developed some new exercises and hands-on techniques that can achieve the same results. My criteria for choosing the exercises and techniques were that they must be effective for improving the function of the social engagement nervous system for most people; they must be easy to learn; and they must be easy to do.

I was blessed with good intuitions—the exercises and hands-on techniques that I present in this book actually do work to bring most people into a state of social engagement, and most people can easily learn them from this book.

ALMOST EVERYONE CAN BENEFIT FROM THESE EXERCISES

This book is mainly written for average people—not necessarily just health care professionals—and for anyone who has failed to find satisfactory solutions to their health needs within existing treatment modalities. The book can also be a resource for psychologists, psychiatrists, hands-on body therapists, physicians, and other health care practitioners who are looking for new ways to bring about positive changes in their clients. This approach can be used as an alternative or as complementary to other types of treatments.

Many of us have a hard time affording the rising costs of medical treatment, or want to avoid the negative side effects that can come from medicines. The techniques and exercises in this book are a safe and inexpensive form of self-help. Once you have bought this book, the treatments are free!

Warning: If you are taking medicine prescribed by a physician and want to reduce your dosage or stop taking the medicine entirely, please initiate a process of cooperation with your doctor. Do not change your dosage or stop taking your medicine without consulting them.

These exercises should in no way replace medical care by a physician, but they will, I hope, help you to become healthier.

The Healing Power of the Polyvagal Theory

A variety of very different health issues are partly caused by vagus nerve dysfunction. Following are case stories of successful treatments that I have given for specific issues, including respiratory difficulties (such as COPD), migraine headaches, and autism-spectrum disorders.

These stories give you a sense of the possibilities that the Polyvagal Theory opens up for health care. Later in the book, I will present other cases from a wider range of more general physical and psychological problems, including stress, depression, and various psychiatric diagnoses. These cases, based on my understanding of the Polyvagal Theory, involved the application of hands-on techniques that I used to bring about a state of ventral vagal activity.

Rather than encouraging readers to rely on treatment by a therapist, I have developed extremely simple self-help exercises for this book that achieve the same results. A non-trained reader can learn most or all of the self-help exercises by carefully digesting the information in these pages. These methods of treatment are both effective and safe. You can use these exercises and apply these techniques to achieve similar positive results to help yourself and others.

If you are a therapist in a clinical setting, you would first test the other person's autonomic nervous system; then you can demonstrate and teach the self-help exercises. Afterward, you should test again to make sure that you have achieved the desired changes. You can suggest that your client use these self-help exercises in the future if necessary.

Relieving COPD and Hiatal Hernia

Though many people have heard about COPD (chronic obstructive pulmonary disease) only relatively recently, it is one of the world's most common non-communicable health problems. COPD is a disease state characterized by chronically poor airflow, shortness of breath, and coughing. People with this problem cannot exert themselves physically and have increasing difficulty breathing.

It is currently believed that COPD has many causes, including smoking and exposure to environmental toxins, in reaction to which the body creates a surplus of fibers that block the airways in the bronchioles and lungs. This blockage of the airways is assumed to be the cause of the individual's breathing difficulties.

It is often difficult for those with COPD to remain actively employed and to maintain their previous lifestyles, so they often have difficulty planning ahead in terms of financial commitments. They often also have difficulty maintaining their activity levels outside of work, and therefore have a reduced quality of life.[49]

Although steroids and inhalers can temporarily improve breathing, the problems can return as soon as the medicine wears off. And inhalers and steroids often have negative side effects if used over a long period of time, so they are generally recommended for short-term use only. Furthermore, most people around the world with COPD cannot afford inhalers and steroids and therefore do not have access to them. The bottom line is that there is no known cure for their condition, which steadily worsens until they succumb to an early death.

COPD typically worsens over time until the respiration is so limited that it cannot sustain life. People with COPD, accordingly, have a reduced life expectancy. Worldwide, COPD affects 329 million people, or nearly 5 percent of the population, although the true prevalence may be higher due to underdiagnosis. In 2012, COPD ranked as the third-leading cause of death (after heart disease and cancer), killing more than three million people.[50]

How is it possible that, in spite of spending trillions of dollars on medical research every year, we are still unable to successfully treat this widespread illness? Are we looking for answers in the wrong places? As far as I know, until now there has been no known successful treatment for COPD.

Perhaps there are solutions that are not based on drugs or surgery. From my success with the following case, among others, I have come to believe that many underlying problems with COPD stem from autonomic nervous system dysfunction, and that COPD is an example of a health issue that might be addressed successfully using the insights gained from the Polyvagal Theory.

Doctors and hospitals do more elaborate and expensive testing than ever before, but they usually overlook evaluating the function of the autonomic nervous system. This is unfortunate, because patients can be screened quickly and inexpensively for ventral vagus branch function— which affects many other body functions.

Restoring the function of the vagus nerve is a key element of my successful treatment of COPD. In my clinic I have been able to help most COPD-diagnosed patients to improve their breathing in spite of the accepted belief in the medical community that no medical treatment can effectively improve a person's mechanical ventilation.

By getting the autonomic nervous system to function better, I have been able to help people with a wide variety of chronic problems that have not been helped by other modalities of treatment, whether allopathic or alternative. Although I have worked with many different kinds of health issues, I was especially pleased by my successes in helping COPD-diagnosed clients to improve their breathing capacity. Through a combination of my hands-on treatments and their own practice of self-help exercises, they were able to improve their breathing capacity and thereby increase oxygen uptake into their blood.

COPD AND HIATAL HERNIA: A CASE STUDY

Although I do not have the facilities to measure vital capacity accurately in my clinic, one of my clients who was diagnosed with COPD had been measured at the hospital before he started with me, and again after seven sessions. His vital capacity (a test for lung function) had improved from 70 percent to 102 percent. (Vital capacity is measured against the average of other people of one's age group, calibrated by body weight. It is possible for a person to be above the average for people in the same age group and calibrated for weight. Therefore it is possible for a person to have a vital capacity of more than 100 percent.)

This client's original lung and bronchial scans showed white areas that the doctors assumed were a concentration of extra fibers, which were supposed to be part of the reason why he was not absorbing sufficient oxygen. My belief was that if we improved the movement of his lungs as he breathed, in time the extra fibers might be absorbed. I saw this client again recently, and his absorption of oxygen had improved by 15 percent.

My clinic is in a building in a charming old neighborhood in Copenhagen. There is no elevator, and my office is one flight up. One day I was expecting a new client, a forty-four-year-old man with difficulty breathing. He had told me in an earlier phone conversation that he had a medical diagnosis of COPD.

When I heard a knock at the door, I opened it and saw him at the top of the stairs, clutching the railing tightly with one hand, gasping rapidly, and fighting for his next breath. He said that he had had to stop twice to catch his breath on the way up.

Before he developed this problem, this man had been in great physical shape. He had actively participated in various sports; his special passion was cross-country skiing. He had just returned from a skiing vacation in the Swiss Alps with his two children, but this time he did not get onto skis; he had to sit on the terrace at the restaurant, wrapped in a blanket, watching them come down the slope without him.

He told me about the several large white areas in his lung scan, indicating the growth of extra fibers, which the doctors had told him were the cause of his difficulty breathing. I could not deny the fact that there were white areas on the scan, but I did not buy into their explanation that these fibers were the only cause of his breathing difficulties. I looked at his problem as a muscular-skeletal issue: if I could get his ribs and respiratory diaphragm to move more normally, I was sure that his breathing would improve, even if scans and x-rays still showed the existence of those extra fibers.

From many years of clinical experience, I had come to suspect that when there is a dysfunction in a visceral organ—in this case the lungs— the cause might partly stem from a dysfunction in the autonomic nervous system nerves serving that organ. The ventral and dorsal branches of the vagus nerve, as well as the sympathetic nervous system, innervate the heart and lungs. The dorsal vagus also provides the primary pathways to the subdiaphragmatic vagus nerve branch that extends to the visceral organs below the diaphragm.

The dorsal branch of the vagus nerve constricts the bronchioles, reducing airflow. The sympathetic nervous system (associated with stress) dilates the bronchioles, allowing the maximum flow of air. When the ventral branch of the vagus nerve functions properly, the bronchioles relax, allowing an adequate flow of air to and from the lungs.

Before I started treating this short-of-breath cross-country skier, I asked him where he felt movement when he breathed. He replied that he lifted his upper chest on the inbreath and that it settled back down on the outbreath. I could see what he was describing—he was almost panting, and his breathing was shallow, rapid, and high in his chest.

However, this chest movement did not result from lifting of the respiratory diaphragm. Rather, it came from the muscles in his neck and shoulders tightening in order to lift his upper ribs. Over time, these tensions had pulled his head into a forward posture (more on this later), which further restricted his breathing.

I stood behind him and placed both of my hands lightly on the sides of the lower part of his chest, sensing whether there was any movement in his lowest two ribs. When the respiratory diaphragm functions properly, it tightens on the inbreath, pushing downward and laterally expanding the lower two ribs. The man had only a minimal amount of lateral rib movement on his right side, and no detectable lateral movement on the left side.

I like my clients to participate in the evaluation of their own breathing by noticing where there is movement in their chest and belly. Then they can participate by evaluating whether there are any positive changes as a result of my treatment. I showed this client where to feel the movement of different parts of his chest when he breathed in. I asked him what, if any, movement of his ribs he could feel out to the sides. He said that he could not feel any movement.

I tested the function of the ventral branch of his vagus nerve. (I describe how to do this test in Chapter 4.) It took me less than thirty seconds to determine that the ventral branch of his vagus nerve was dysfunctional. Would there be any improvement in his breathing from establishing good function in his ventral vagus with the Basic Exercise?

I asked this client to lie down on his back on my massage table, and taught him how to do the Basic Exercise. (You can find instructions for this exercise and others in Part Two.) My cross-country skier had an immediate improvement in his respiration; he was breathing more slowly, more deeply, and without strain. His ribs were expanding out to the sides as he inhaled—he could feel this himself. This represented a major improvement for someone suffering from COPD who had difficulty breathing. I again tested the function of the ventral branch of his vagus nerve, and found that it was now working as it should.

Medical doctors and researchers often use a spirometer to test lung capacity. People tend to get nervous, however, when they think that they are being tested, causing them to tense up and restrict their breathing. I prefer to evaluate breathing functionally. I began with the observation that this client had a very difficult time climbing one flight of stairs, indicating how his breathing was impaired when he had to exert himself in a normal, everyday situation.

After the treatment, my client looked much more relaxed. When he stood up, I could see that he breathed more deeply and more slowly, and that he had better color in his face. He told me that he felt much better. Not bad for less than six minutes—an examination, one exercise, and a reexamination.

My next goal was to further improve the movement of his respiratory diaphragm. The lateral movement of his ribs on the right side had increased, but there was still almost no palpable lateral movement of the lower ribs on his left side. By comparing his right side with his left, I clearly felt that something on his left side was interfering with the movement of his diaphragm. From my experience with many patients, I suspected that this might be caused by a hiatal hernia.

What is a hiatal hernia? The stomach is on the left side of the abdomen, normally below the respiratory diaphragm. The esophagus—the elastic muscular tube that connects the back of the mouth to the top of the stomach—passes through a round opening (hiatus) in the respiratory diaphragm. The ventral branch of the vagus nerve innervates the upper third of the esophagus, allowing its muscle fibers to change their length and lift or lower the stomach, although the typical medical understanding of a hiatal hernia does not consider the role of the vagus nerve.

If there is good vagal function, the esophagus can relax and lengthen, letting the stomach move down slightly into the abdomen as the diaphragm tightens on the inbreath. Ideally, as the diaphragm ascends and descends freely along the esophagus, the contents of the chest remain in the chest (above the diaphragm), and the contents of the abdomen remain in the abdomen (below the diaphragm). However, in cases of vagal dysfunction, the upper third of the esophagus tightens and shortens, pulling the stomach up against the bottom of the respiratory diaphragm. (See "Stomach 2" in the Appendix.)

In extreme cases, the esophagus can be so tight and short that it pulls the stomach up against the diaphragm, forcing its opening to enlarge and pulling part of the stomach up into the chest. This is called a hiatal hernia. (The word *hiatus* means "gap or interruption," and a hernia is a protrusion through an opening in tissue.)

In addition to major difficulties breathing, people with hiatal hernias often have acid reflux. When stomach acid comes up and burns the esophagus or back of the throat, the result is acid reflux, also called GERD (gastroesophageal reflux disease), or heartburn. Other symptoms can include a bloated feeling after eating, and a propensity to eat several small meals rather than three normal meals daily.

Normal breathing should involve the diaphragm moving up and down (see "Diaphragmatic Breathing" on page 101). In cases of breathing difficulties such as asthma and cold lungs (a.k.a. COPD), I have found the shortened esophagus to be a factor that disrupts normal breathing—in fact, I believe it is at the core of many breathing disorders. When the stomach is pulled up into it, the diaphragm cannot descend freely on the inbreath.

When I treat the vagus nerve with the Basic Exercise and then use a technique adapted from visceral osteopathy to lengthen and relax the esophagus, breathing difficulties disappear immediately, and the client breathes deeply without effort. That's often all it takes!

Treating a Hiatal Hernia

Following is an osteopathic visceral-massage technique for treatment of a hiatal hernia. It works well as a simple self-help exercise.

I first instruct clients how to do the Basic Exercise (see Part Two). Then I use a simple osteopathic technique to pull their stomach down and to stretch (lengthen) and relax the esophagus. I usually teach them to do this for themselves. With this protocol, I have helped many patients with diagnoses such as asthma, pulmonary fibrosis, and shortness of breath.

The stomach is on the left side of the abdomen, just under the rib cage. Place the fingertips of one hand lightly on the top of where you imagine you can find the stomach. The stomach is soft but palpable. You should be able to feel the stomach if you slowly and gently extend your fingertips into the abdominal muscles. You only want to feel the top surface of the stomach. Under no circumstances should your move be painful. If the person experiences pain, you should stop immediately. Gently pull it downward toward the feet until you sense the first sign of resistance— usually after pulling it only about one half-inch to one inch (Figure 1). Hold it at that point of slight resistance until the esophagus relaxes. Although you might be tempted to push the stomach down in order to stretch the esophagus, it in not necessary to exert any force. If you have your fingers on the top of the stomach, you will signal the nerves for the esophagus to lengthen, and the stomach will descend in the abdomen, making room for the respiratory diaphragm to descend on the inbreath.

A sigh or a swallow usually accompanies this moment of relaxation. At this point, it feels as if the muscular resistance to the stomach's being pulled down melts. And immediately the person is able to breathe more easily and deeply.

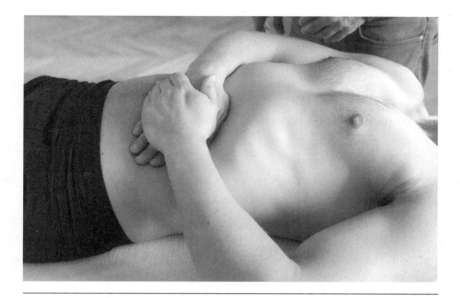

Figure 1. Hiatal hernia treatment

For this particular client, I guided him in this simple self-help technique so that, by gently pulling his stomach downward, he was able to stretch his esophagus and breathe more freely. With a relaxed esophagus, his stomach was free to move into a better position, lower in his abdomen, an inch or two below his respiratory diaphragm. His diaphragm could then move freely up and down, sliding normally over the outer surface of his esophagus, now that there was room for it to descend on the inbreath. His lower ribs could also expand laterally to both sides. His breathing was much deeper, and markedly slower. He was exchanging a greater volume of air on every breath.

Now came the functional test: The landing at my office door is one flight up from street level, and I asked my client to go up to the top of the stairwell—another four flights up—and then to come back down again. When he returned, he was breathing hard, but his breathing was deeper. Smiling, he said, "I ran the whole way up and the whole way down. I didn't need to stop once." This was a man who could not walk up one flight of stairs without stopping to catch his breath before our session.

This client continues to take occasional sessions with me. In addition to treating his hiatal hernia, we addressed tensions in other visceral organs that can also hamper breathing. He continued doing the Basic Exercise, the self-help technique for hiatal hernia, and other visceral-massage techniques. I also gave him some movement exercises. After twelve weeks, he was able to ride a bike for several hours with his brother, who had been a national triathlon champion in Denmark. When I last spoke with him, his breathing was continuing to improve, and he was planning a biking trip in the mountains of Switzerland with his brother. This was only six months after he started his sessions with me.

When this man was medically scanned again, there were still white areas in his lungs, showing the continued presence of fibers. However, the fibers did not seem to be restricting his breathing. The fibers do reduce the effectiveness of lung tissue in absorbing oxygen. But with a far greater lung capacity, he was now able to perform at a higher level than many athletes.

I believe most attempts to treat COPD have been using the wrong map, failing to take into account that part of the problem can be traced to dysfunction of the vagus nerve. I believe that the cause of COPD often involves a lack of activity in the ventral branch of the vagus nerve, leaving the dorsal branch's activity unchecked.

The dorsal branch constricts the bronchioles, making it difficult to get enough air into the lungs. This constriction is appropriate for the immobilized state of shutdown, for instance, in a crocodile after it has eaten a big meal and must lie still in order to digest. However, if this constriction is unchecked, it becomes problematic for humans trying to function normally in everyday life.

Using the Basic Exercise to activate the function of the ventral branch of the vagus nerve moves people out of the dorsal-branch state of shutdown, so that their bronchioles are no longer constricted.

The Basic Exercise, combined with stretching of the esophagus, takes only a few minutes. There is no prescription medicine required, and it is immediately effective, with no negative side effects. To me, this is evidence that the widely accepted explanation of the cause of COPD is not the whole story. The man that I treated brought me x-rays and scans showing white areas in his lungs, and had been told that these areas were fibers causing breathing restrictions. If after ten minutes of my treatment he was able to breathe more normally, the idea that his breathing was restricted by the fibers does not hold—or at least we can say that this was not the only explanation.

For this man with COPD, improving the function of his ventral vagus nerve, bringing his head back from a forward position, and easing the function of his respiratory diaphragm contributed to improvement in his vital capacity. This was confirmed by hospital tests.

Diaphragmatic Breathing

Good diaphragmatic breathing is an important element of social engagement. Every person I have observed in my clinic who is in a state of stress or dorsal vagal activity has a disturbed pattern of breathing.

Normal breathing should involve up-and-down movement of the diaphragm. In order to evaluate whether this is happening, I place my hands lightly on the sides of the chest at the level of the last two ribs. If there is diaphragmatic breathing, I can detect a lateral movement of the lower two ribs on both sides. However, if there is a hiatal hernia, I can feel lateral movement on the right side but almost none on the left.

When we cannot inhale with a normal lowering of their respiratory diaphragm, we find alternative ways to make space for the expanding lungs. One very common way is to lift the shoulders and upper ribs. This is called high costal breathing ("costal" refers to ribs). This breathing pattern is associated with the emotions of fear, anxiety, and panic.

Another common pattern in non-diaphragmatic breathing is to inhale using the abdominal muscles. Sometimes, when we are typically short of breath, the belly is distended, soft, and flabby. The belly muscles are too soft, and when they go slack the intestines descend, pulling the lungs down. Sometimes people call this "belly breathing" and interpret it as a good sign because they can see that the breath is going down into the abdomen. However, it does not actively involve tightening the respiratory diaphragm. People breathing this way often hold their stomach muscles tight on the inbreath. The muscles of their abdomen feel hard. This breathing pattern is associated with anger.

Ideally, the abdomen and chest expand and contract rhythmically, at the same time. The lower two ribs (R11 and R12) move to the sides, down, and back with expansion. The next five ribs up (R6–R10) swing out to the sides; this lateral movement is likened to that of a "bucket handle." The next group of ribs above those (R5 to R1) lifts straight upward, along with the sternum, in a movement described as the "pump handle."

If we lose optimal tonus in our diaphragm, we also lose proper tonus in our entire musculoskeletal system. We tend to collapse into our body, and exhibit the breathing of someone who is shut down and manifesting depressive behavior. If, on the other hand, we tighten the diaphragm and push it down onto our gut, we get the body and breathing of someone in a state of anger.

The vagus nerve has both sensory and motor fibers that affect and are affected by the movements of respiration. There are four times as many sensory (afferent, or inward-transmitting) nerve fibers in the respiratory branch of the vagus nerve as there are motor (efferent, or outward-transmitting) nerves, and these are constantly monitoring the functioning of the respiratory diaphragm.

Proper function of the motor fibers of the ventral vagus is necessary to facilitate relaxed, efficient breathing. When the respiratory diaphragm is not working properly and does not descend on the inbreath, we use muscles activated by either our spinal sympathetic chain or our dorsal vagal circuit, so a breathing pattern that fails to make proper use of the diaphragm will communicate through the sensory nerve fibers that we are threatened or in danger. This is one example of how feedback from sensory branches of cranial nerves influences the state of our autonomic nervous system.

Shoulder, Neck, and Head Pain:
CN XI, Trapezius, and SCM

In addition to being one of the five "social engagement" nerves, cranial nerve XI (the "spinal accessory nerve") has a special muscular function. It innervates the trapezius and the sternocleidomastoid (SCM), two large muscles in the neck and shoulder. (See "Trapezius" and "Sternocleido-mastoid" in the Appendix.) These are the only skeletal muscles below the face and head that are not innervated by spinal nerves. If either of these two muscles is chronically either tense or flaccid, it will respond differently to massage treatment and movement training than any other muscle of the body.

Shoulder problems are among the most common forms of musculo-skeletal problems. Dysfunction in CN XI often leads to pain and stiffness in the neck and shoulders, and sometimes simply improving the function of CN X and CN XI with the Basic Exercise is enough to eliminate pain or restricted movement in this area. After doing the exercise, we might want to try other ways to treat other problems stemming from these muscles; for example, see the self-help treatment for migraine headaches described in Part Two. Doing the Basic Exercise seems to also instantaneously improve the function of all five nerves necessary for social engagement for most people.

Returning to the trapezius and sternocleidomastoid muscles, we note that dysfunction of CN XI and/or a lack of proper tonus in the trapezius and SCM muscles are involved in many other health issues besides neck and shoulder pain and stiffness. These include migraines, forward head posture, breathing difficulties, chronic spinal sympathetic chain activation, chronic dorsal vagal state, and shortened life expectancy.

The trapezius and SCM are also determining factors in the shape and health of the spine. Furthermore, a chronic tension in the sternocleido-mastoid muscles on one side can actually change the shape of the back of the head, leaving it flat on one side because of the constant pull of the muscle on the temporal bones (the skull plates behind the ears). In every child I've treated on the autism spectrum, I have observed this distortion in the shape of the back of their head.[51] (See Part Two for a technique to round the back of the head.)

Turning the head to either side should be an even, well-coordinated movement, without stops or jerks, and without deviation from a smooth curve. The head should be able to turn ninety degrees, or slightly more.

People often complain about reduced range of movement, stiffness, or pain in their neck and shoulders when they rotate their head to one side. If the pain or stiffness is on the side opposite to the direction in which they turn their head, the shoulder problem is most likely either the trapezius or the sternocleidomastoid muscle on the side toward which they are turning. If the pain is on the same side as the turn, the problem is not cranial nerve XI and the trapezius and SCM but is most likely due to the *levator scapulae*. In Part Two there is a set of exercises called "The Salamander Exercises," which improve the neck's capacity for lateral movement. This exercise can be slightly painful at first, but if we are persistent, we can increase the range of movement, improve the flow of blood to CN XI, and improve the function of our trapezius and sternocleidomastoid muscles.

The *Levator Scapulae* Muscle

We can improve the function of the cranial nerves, and improve the rotation of the head to the right and left, with the Basic Exercise and the Salamander Exercises. But these still might not be enough to allow full freedom in the turning of the head, since many other muscles of the neck are involved in head movement, and tension in any of them can restrict head turning.

If we have pain in our neck on the same side our head is turning toward, then the problem is not cranial nerve XI and the trapezius and SCM. It is most likely coming from another muscle, the *levator scapulae* ("shoulder-blade lifter"). In these cases, working on cranial nerve XI and the trapezius and sternocleidomastoid muscles will probably not remove all of the pain and stiffness.

Janet Travell, David Simons, and Lois Simons, in their book *Myofascial Pain and Dysfunction: The Trigger Point Manual,* nicknamed the *levator scapulae* the "Stiff Neck" muscle.[52] This pair of muscles reaches down from the top vertebrae to the shoulder blade, along either side of the neck.

I have found that directly massaging the *levator scapulae* gives relief, but only temporarily—the muscle dysfunction quickly returns. The problem is probably that the *levator scapulae* is undertoned. So if you want a more lasting result, Tom Myers suggested massaging the supraspinatus muscle (along the top of the shoulder blade) to improve the tonus of the *levator scapulae.* (See "Supraspinatus" in the Appendix.)

Benjamin Shield suggested another approach. He observed that with a side-bending of the upper cervical vertebrae, you can open the spaces between C1 and C3 to take the pressure off of the spinal nerves that go to the *levator scapulae.* You might try the upper part (Level 1) of the Salamander Exercises, tipping the head to one side to open the spaces between C1 and C3.

THE TRAPEZIUS AND STERNOCLEIDOMASTOID MUSCLES

Problems with the trapezius and sternocleidomastoid muscles are more serious than just the discomforts of pain, stiffness, or migraines. Usually people with dysfunction in either of these two muscles are not socially engaged, and they are prone to all of the problems that I earlier described as the "heads of the Hydra" (see the beginning of Part One). Correcting the function of these two muscles usually improves the function of CN XI and can restore the state of social engagement.

Because these two muscles are innervated by a cranial nerve, they are different from the other 660 skeletal muscles in the rest of the body, which are all innervated by spinal nerves. Tension in any of these other muscles can cause pain, reduced range of movement, and stiffness. Dysfunction in the sternocleidomastoid and trapezius muscles, by contrast, is related to a host of serious health issues that we usually do not associate with muscular problems.

The trapezius muscles are a pair of thin, flat, trapezoid-shaped, super-ficial muscles covering a large area of the back of the neck, shoulders, and torso. They originate on the occipital bone, at the base of the back of the skull, and attach to the spinous processes of the shoulder blades and the spinous process of each vertebra of the cervical and thoracic spine (in the neck and torso). The sternocleidomastoid (SCM) muscles attach to the tip of the mastoid process of the temporal bones, along the sides of the skull just behind the ears. Then the muscle splits into two "bellies" that wrap diagonally forward and down, with one part attaching to the top of the sternum (breastbone) and the other part to the medial section of the clavicle (collarbone). Because the two muscles' bellies attach at slightly different places on the skull, they pull the head at slightly differ-ent angles. Also, because the sternal and clavicular bellies of the SCM attach in differ-ent locations on the torso, they also contribute to the rotation of the head.

The SCM muscles on both sides muscles can be likened to reins that allow a horseback rider to steer the movement of the horse's head. The rider pulls in the reins on one side while letting out slack on the other side. If there is no chronic tension in our SCM on either side, our head would be perfectly balanced on our neck; it would turn just as easily to the right or to the left without restriction or pain. Our head would come to a natural resting position looking straight ahead.

However, there is often tightness in one of the bellies of the SCM on one side, resulting in a stiff neck. This makes rotation of the neck easy toward one side, but difficult toward the other. Since the SCM is innervated by the eleventh cranial nerve, this stiffness is often caused by a dysfunction of CN XI and is almost always concurrent with a dysfunction of the vagus nerve.

If the bellies of the SCM attaching to the sternum tighten on both sides symmetrically, they will shorten the neck, making it thicker, and pull the head forward. This has been described as a "bull neck." If the bellies of the SCM attaching to the clavicle tighten symmetrically, they pull the head backward, making the neck thinner and longer (a "swan neck").

In her book *Rolfing*,[53] pioneering body therapist Dr. Ida Rolf calls our attention to the fact that the trapezius and the sternocleidomastoid muscles comprise the outer ring of neck muscles. Inside this outer ring, there are many smaller muscles that help us to make finer movements of the head, to lift the upper ribs when we breathe, and to swallow.

The complicated coordination of tension and relaxation of the muscles that turn our head requires precise muscle control. This is programmed into our nervous system in such a way that we do not have to think about the mechanics of it. When something catches our attention, we automatically focus our eyes on it. The movement of our head follows the direction of our eyes, and then the movement of our body follows the movement of our head. The eyes focus on an object of interest, and center it in the visual field; then the eleventh cranial nerve innervates the fibers of the trapezius and SCM muscles in order to turn the head in that direction.

We were born with this ability to coordinate our eye, head, and body movements. When a baby is lying on its stomach, if an object in front of it suddenly moves or changes its speed, the baby's eyes will focus on the object and follow the movement, first with its eyes and then with its head. We respond to sound in the same way. If there is a sound that catches our attention, we move our head to center the sound between our ears. All of this requires complex coordination of the trapezius, SCM, and other muscles.

TRAPEZIUS AND SCM MUSCLES IN ACTION
ON THE SERENGETI PLAIN

A cheetah is the fastest mammal on Earth, able to run at speeds of up to sixty miles per hour. Running at that incredible speed, the cheetah keeps its eyes fixed on the animal it is chasing. The eleventh cranial nerve enables the cheetah to turn its head and, as its head turns, its body follows.

An antelope being chased by the cheetah looks for clear areas where it can get away from the cheetah without bumping into anything. When its eyes find such a space, its head follows the direction of the eyes and then its body follows.

Although it is not as fast as the cheetah, the antelope has an advantage: if it ran in a straight line, the cheetah could easily catch it, but with its light body and thin legs, the antelope can turn faster. So, to avoid being captured by the cheetah, the antelope zigs and zags. The cheetah is unable to do this quite as quickly; because it is so agile, therefore, a healthy adult antelope will usually survive being chased by a cheetah. The antelope also has the endurance to run for a longer period of time and outlast a pursuing cheetah.

When a cheetah, lion, tiger, or other predator chases its prey and does not manage to bring it down right away, it becomes exhausted from the intense effort, and it takes several hours to regain the strength to try again. Therefore, before it exerts itself, the cheetah spends time studying the herd of antelopes in order to pick out one that is injured or old, or a newborn hiding in the long grass near its mother. Half of all antelope fawns are lost to predators before reaching adulthood.

For both the hunter and the hunted, survival depends in part on turning their heads effortlessly, and the muscles primarily responsible for this are the trapezius and the sternocleidomastoid—both innervated by cranial nerve XI. Because turning the head is a matter of life and death, it is not surprising that the structure of CN XI is highly developed and complex, for precise innervation of the individual fibers of these muscles.

USE OF TRAPEZIUS MUSCLES WHEN CRAWLING

The trapezius is one of the very first muscles that we humans use as babies. When a baby lies on its stomach, its first movement is to arch its back and lift its head using its trapezius muscles. Then, with its head up, the baby can turn its head and look around using the sternocleidomastoid muscles. (See "Baby on stomach" in the Appendix.)

The next step in the baby's development will be to lift its head high enough to bring its arms under its shoulders to support the weight of its upper body. With this, the baby will soon be able to come up on all fours. In this position, tensing the fibers of the upper trapezius extends and arches the neck and lifts the head, and the face looks forward. (See "Baby on all fours" in the Appendix.) In order to do this, the baby tenses all the fibers of the three parts of the trapezius more or less equally. The baby arches its lower back with its lower trapezius, pulls the shoulders together with the middle trapezius, and lifts its head up and tips it back with the upper trapezius. In addition to the trapezius muscle, the head is held up and balanced on the vertebrae of the neck partly due to the action of the *semispinalis capitis,* the largest muscle in the posterior neck. Then the sternocleidomastoid muscles can rotate the head quite easily.

At this stage in its development, the baby supports its weight on its hands and knees and moves much like other four-legged mammals. After a short while, the baby can begin to crawl forward, moving with first one arm forward and the other one back. This asymmetrical pattern of arm movement when crawling requires using the trapezius muscles asymmetrically.

With the body supported on all fours, the arms and thighs are at a ninety-degree angle to the trunk. As the baby pushes down with its arms, there is equal force pushing the arm back up into the socket of the shoulder joint, and the proprioceptive nerves in the shoulder joint can report to the brain that the arms and shoulders feel right and are in balance.

CHANGES IN TRAPEZIUS USE WHEN GOING FROM CRAWLING TO STANDING

Human babies support their weight on all fours when they crawl. Human beings have the same physical structure as four-legged animals in terms of the muscles, bones, and nerves involved in this movement.

We live in gravity, and gravity is always pulling us down. When we crawled on all fours, we distributed our weight more or less evenly on our four limbs, which held our weight by pushing up into our body. This is a stable structure.

When we stood up to balance on our hind legs, we had to use our muscles and bones in a completely new way. Everything changed in the balance of tensions in our muscular and skeletal systems. Instead of a more or less even muscle tonus in the muscle fibers, some muscles became chronically tensed, and others became flaccid. Instead of holding our weight on four supports, we balance our heavy upper body entirely on the two ball-and-socket joints between the legs and hips when we stand, which is most unstable compared to a four-legged stance. (See "Baby standing" in the Appendix.)

Over decades, standing on our back legs can give rise to many problems that four-legged animals do not have. Common to most of us is an increase in our forward head posture (FHP) as we age. (See the following section on FHP and its related health problems.)

When we first came up to crawl on all fours, the trapezius muscle held our head up high. The three parts of the trapezius functioned like a single muscle in which all of the fibers had roughly the same tension. Some of the muscle fibers worked to pull the shoulders back and together to support our upper spine, and others fibers pulling in other directions worked to lift the head back and up.

But when we stood up, parts of the trapezius muscle lost their integrity; they were no longer needed to pull our shoulders together in the back and tilt our head up, as before. Rather than acting as a single muscle, these muscle fibers organized themselves into three functional units—now seen as the upper, middle, and lower trapezius—and these three groups of fibers began to work as separate entities. One part, therefore, might be overly tense while another part is under-tensed. This is reflected in the position of the bones of not only the shoulder but the spine as well. (See "Trapezius" in the Appendix.)

The spine of a human being has a much different form than that of a horse, a goat, or a giraffe. A four-legged animal supports part of its weight on its front legs, in contrast to a human being whose arms hang freely from the shoulder joint. There is no longer a pushing of the arms into the shoulder joint.

If we have shoulder pain, we often ask ourselves what we did to create the pain—we must have lifted something heavy, or thrown something, such as a baseball, which we were not used to doing. However, an unrecognized factor in the creation of imbalances leading to shoulder pain might be changes that have occurred because we are standing upright only on our legs. And there is no telling what a lifetime habit of sitting still on chairs does to our musculoskeletal structure. It is not a surprise that many physical therapists report that the most common problems that they treat are shoulder problems.

The human spine has weaknesses that lead to stiff necks, backaches, and shoulder problems. When we stand up, the relationship between the head and the spine changes compared to when we were on all fours. (See "Baby standing" in the Appendix.) In order to balance on our legs, the upper part of the trapezius is no longer positioned to hold the head up and back, and the head tends to slide forward.

The middle part of the trapezius muscle no longer pulls the shoulder blades together toward the spine to make a stable base. Instead, for most of us, our shoulder blades glide down our back, forward, and around to our sides. Compared with the deep barrel chest of a four-legged animal, our upper chest caves in, and our belly hangs out. If an actor assumed this posture, it would be to portray a character who had lost a sense of self-esteem.

When the lower part of the trapezius does not function as it used to when we were crawling on all fours, our spine shortens, and our head moves into a forward position. These changes are not due to increased muscular tension but rather to a general loss of a balanced tonus in the three parts of the trapezius muscle that used to hold our head up against the constant pull of gravity.

To improve the function of the trapezius muscle, therefore, we need to improve the tonus of the muscle fibers in all three parts of the trapezius by stimulating the nerves to the muscle. We can do that with a simple movement that I call the "Twist and Turn Exercise" (see Part Two). Unlike most other exercises, this exercise neither stretches nor strengthens the muscle; by tightening and releasing muscle tension, it simply wakes up the nerves innervating the trapezius muscle. Overly tense areas of the muscle can relax, while muscle tone increases in areas that need it.

ASYMMETRY IN TRAPEZIUS MUSCLE TENSION

There are always differences in tension among the groups of fibers comprising the upper, middle, and lower trapezius muscles. There is also a difference between the right and left sides. This asymmetry of the various parts can disrupt the balance in the two shoulders.

Because the trapezius attaches to the cervical and thoracic spine, imbalances in tension between the right and left trapezius muscles add to rotations, extensions, flexions, and side-bending of the thoracic vertebrae. This changes the internal space within the chest, which in turn affects the function of the heart and lungs.

In some cases this asymmetry can also compress the spinal nerves exiting from these segments, affecting the organs they serve. Some of the spinal nerves (T1–T4) go to the heart, and some (T5–T8) to the lungs. Others (T9 and below) connect to various visceral organs.

ASYMMETRY IN STERNOCLEIDOMASTOID TENSION

The sternocleidomastoid muscles on both sides are the primary muscles for turning the head left and right, and chronic or acute tension in a sternocleidomastoid muscle results in a stiff neck. A baby with this issue tends to turn its head to one side when lying on its back. As the child gets older, this condition might be diagnosed as torticollis ("twisted neck").

If you examine the back of the head of someone with a stiff neck, you may find it to be flat on one side. If so, the same technique described in the "Technique for Rounding a Flat Back of the Head" on page 178 might not only relax a tight sternocleidomastoid muscle but also to some degree start to round the back of the head, even in an adult.

A stiff neck usually accompanies a rotation of the first cervical vertebra, called the atlas (see "Atlas" in the Appendix), resulting in a reduced blood flow to the brainstem. In adults, a stiff neck may indicate dysfunction of the eleventh cranial nerve which, as noted earlier, is one of the five cranial nerves necessary for social engagement. So releasing SCM tension often makes it easier for us to be socially engaged.

This observation is not new; we find references that go back thousands of years. There are surprisingly many references to "stiff-necked" people in the Bible. An example from Nehemiah 9:17 says: "They refused to listen, and did not remember the wonders you performed among them.

They became stiff-necked, and in their rebellion they appointed a leader to return to their slavery in Egypt."

A NEW PICTURE OF CN XI

Turning the head is one of the most important and complex movements of the body. It is one of the first movements that a baby makes, and we are so familiar with this movement that we usually do not even think about it. Control of the trapezius and SCM muscles requires a coordinated tensing and relaxation of their many individual muscle fibers, and this action depends on a well-functioning CN XI.

Most anatomical illustrations of CN XI attempt to show all the branches of this nerve in a single drawing, but I have personally found those drawings to be confusing. In order to help you gain a clear understanding of the complexity of structure of CN XI, I asked my illustrator to make some new drawings in color that show the three parts of this important cranial nerve. (See the "CN XI" series in the Appendix.) One branch of CN XI originates in the brainstem and used to be called the "cranial division." It is now considered to be a part of the vagus nerve— the branch that innervates the pharyngeal muscles discussed in Chapter 4. Another branch, called the "spinal accessory nerve," exits the spinal cord in the neck just below the cranium before going directly to the fibers of the trapezius and sternocleidomastoid muscles. There is yet another branch of the spinal accessory nerve, made of up nerve branches that leave the spinal cord, weave together, extend up into the cranium through the foramen magnum, reach across the floor of the skull, and then exit through the jugular foramen in the base of the skull.

In spite of their diverse pathways, all the branches of CN XI function together in a coordinated way to innervate the various parts of the trapezius and sternocleidomastoid muscles.

CN XI and the ventral vagus (CN X) are closely linked, not only functionally, through their role as two of the five cranial nerves necessary for social engagement, but structurally. In two of the CN XI drawings in the Appendix, a clear connection can be seen between branches of CN XI and the ventral branch of the vagus nerve after they exit the skull through the jugular foramen: fibers from CN XI intermingle with fibers of the vagus nerve outside the cranium for a few millimeters. In addition to the mixing of their nerve fibers after they exit the jugular foramen, both CN XI and the ventral vagus branch originate in the *nucleus ambiguus,* a strip of nerve fibers in the brainstem.

Therefore, it is not surprising that the function/dysfunction of the vagus nerve is directly mirrored in the function/dysfunction of CN XI. The test for CN XI gives the same results in terms of indicating function/ dysfunction as do tests for the ventral branch of CN X.

CN XI AND THE VENTRAL VAGUS BRANCH

The Trap Squeeze Test for CN XI gives us an indication of the function/ dysfunction of not only CN XI but also the other four nerves necessary for social engagement. All five of these nerves work together; if one is dysfunctional, the others will also be dysfunctional. If we improve the function of one, we also improve the function of the other four.

When I started using the Trap Squeeze Test for CN XI and ventral vagus nerve function by asking my patients to open their mouth and say "ah-ah-ah," I began to notice that whenever there was a difference in tension between the trapezius muscles on the two sides, there was always a dysfunction in the ventral vagus as indicated by the uvular lift test. I decided to carry out an informal study in my clinic.

I tested the next eighty people who came to me for treatment: first I tested their ventral vagus (with the uvular-lift test for vagal pharyngeal- branch function described in Chapter 4), and then their CN XI (with the Trap Squeeze Test). I found a 100 percent correlation between the results of these two tests. On the basis of that, I felt safe concluding that testing the trapezius muscles is a valid indicator of vagal function/ dysfunction.

After clients did the Basic Exercise, I tested them again both ways, and found improvement in both CN XI and the ventral branch of the vagus nerve. The patients agreed with me: "Now, when you squeeze, the two sides feel more like each other." I asked them to turn their head, and to explore the sensations in their head, neck, and shoulders. In almost all cases, they had better movement and could turn their head further, with less or no pain.

The Trap Squeeze Test for Shoulder and Neck Problems

Some of the most common complaints among clients of physical therapists and body therapists involve stiffness in the neck and pain in the shoulder. As discussed above, these problems usually include a lack of proper tonus of the trapezius and/or sternocleidomastoid muscles, either of which may be chronically tense or flaccid.

Most physical therapists, massage therapists, and body therapists start their treatment by working directly on tight shoulder muscles, without considering the state of the client's autonomic nervous system. When people come to my practice with shoulder problems, I base my approach to this on the research findings of Cottingham, Porges, and Lyon.[54]

As suggested by their research, in order to achieve positive results with fascial release, myofascial release, or release of muscle tensions in general, it is important to have a well-functioning ventral vagus nerve before attempting any other intervention. So I first test the ventral branch of the vagus nerve, or use the following test for CN XI function. This test often takes less time, and is less intrusive than my test for vagal function, in which clients have to open their mouths and say "ah-ah-ah" while I use a flashlight to observe uvula-area movement.

For this test, we only have to squeeze the muscles on the top of the shoulder. The Trap Squeeze Test takes only a few seconds, and is well suited for use on children and people on the autism spectrum, with whom we might otherwise encounter difficulties in getting their cooperation for the usual technique.

To use this form of testing, you first need to practice on several people in order to develop the necessary kinesthetic skills. It is normal to feel uncertain the first few times that you try testing the trapezius muscles. However, you will likely find that you can get the feel of it after a few attempts.

CN XI can be tested by sliding, lifting, and rolling the top of the trapezius muscles (on the tops of the shoulders, halfway to the neck), and comparing them on the left and right sides. Although the trapezius muscle covers a large area, it is very thin.

1. Take hold of the trapezius muscle on each side, squeezing it lightly between your thumb and your first finger (Figure 2). Whereas most novices simply grab the muscle, the lighter you squeeze, the better.

2. If you squeeze lightly and slowly, you should be able to lift the muscle slightly away from the underlying muscles.

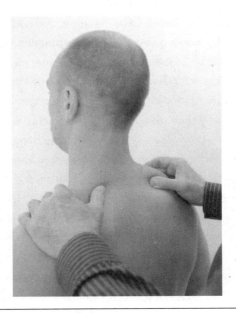

Figure 2. Trap squeeze test

3. Compare the tonus of the trapezius muscle on one side with the tonus of the trapezius muscle on the other side. Do the two sides feel the same to you, or is one side harder than the other? Ideally, both sides should be soft and elastic. However, one side is often soft and

elastic, while the other is not. If you squeeze them slowly, with a light pressure, you can feel that the muscle on one side remains relaxed, soft, and pliable if you push deeper into it, while the other side may react to your squeeze by tensing up and feeling hard, even though you are using a very light pressure.

4. I ask the person who I am testing, "When I squeeze, do the two sides feel the same to you, or do they feel different?" If the person answers that they feel different, I ask, "Which side is more tense?" Here is something that I do not understand, but I encounter it often: more than half the time that I do this test, I disagree with the person I am testing as to which side is more tense, or "harder." I do not know why this is so. But I have come to the conclusion that it does not matter in terms of the success of my treatment; the main point is that my client and I agree that there is a difference between the two sides.

5. If we agree that there is a difference, I take this as an indication of dysfunction in CN XI, and I conclude that their autonomic nervous system is not socially engaged, and that they are in a state of either stress or dorsal vagal withdrawal. We can then take the appropriate steps to restore ventral vagal function before proceeding with any further therapeutic techniques.

Health Problems Related to Forward Head Posture

Serious health problems can stem from kyphosis, or forward head posture (FHP), which is related to dysfunctional trapezius and sternocleidomastoid muscles (Figure 3). A forward head posture is one result of poor posture in general.

As we get older, many of us lose the good posture that we enjoyed as children; we may have increased difficulty breathing and be bothered by occasional dizziness. These issues are generally not considered to be medical problems; doctors tend to assume that they are a natural part of growing older and that nothing can be done about them. There is no medicine or operation to help remedy these conditions as such.

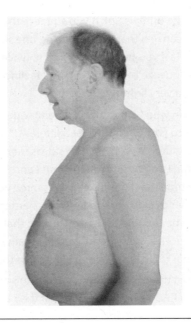

Figure 3. Forward head position

The neck has a tendency to sag when we have FHP, allowing our head to thrust forward. Our upper chest collapses, reducing the space for the heart and lungs. The forward head posture also blocks the action of the muscles responsible for helping to lift the first rib during inhalation, resulting in difficulty breathing.

As time goes on and FHP gets worse, we lose an increasing portion of our breathing capacity. FHP is often found in people with breathing problems such as asthma and COPD.[55] It is no wonder that they experience general fatigue and low levels of energy. Research published in the *Journal of the American Geriatric Society* also reports that they also have shorter life expectancy—shorter even than people who smoke a pack of cigarettes a day—and that older patients with FHP have a significantly higher mortality rate.[56]

Could restrictions in the function of these nerves also be contributing factors in Alzheimer's disease, dementia, and senility?

In addition to reducing breathing capacity, the loss of internal chest space puts pressure on the heart and crowds the blood vessels that go to and from the heart. FHP also compresses the spaces between the vertebrae of the neck and upper thorax, putting pressure on the spinal nerves of the neck and the upper thoracic spine.

Furthermore, forward head posture compresses the vertebral arteries that carry blood up to the head, diminishing blood supply to the face, parts of the brain, and the brainstem, where the social-engagement cranial nerves V, VII, IX, X, and XI originate. When this occurs, as we might expect, we look pale, lack spontaneous facial expression, and are not socially engaged. If these five cranial nerves do not receive adequate blood circulation, they can fail to function properly, and we are likely to be in a state of chronic stress or dorsal vagal activity.

Many aches, pains, and stiffnesses develop over time due to deteriorating posture. According to a Mayo Clinic newsletter, "Forward head posture leads to long-term muscle strain, herniated discs, arthritis, and pinched nerves."[57]

Neurosurgeon and Nobel Prize recipient Dr. Alf Breig stated, "Loss of the cervical curve stretches the spinal cord 5–7 cm and causes disease."[58] The characteristic stiffening of the neck in FHP also stiffens the entire spine. According to Dr. Roger Sperry, Nobel Prize recipient for brain research, "Ninety percent of the stimulation and nutrition to the brain is generated by the movement of the spine."[59]

People with kyphosis often have difficulty breathing, mild back pain, and tenderness and stiffness in the spine. Emotionally, they may experience apathy and indifference about what is happening—also symptomatic of dorsal vagal withdrawal.

Viewed from the side, our ear should be directly above the midline of our shoulder. However, as we age, many of us succumb to a forward head posture, and you can see that the ear has moved forward in relationship to the center of the shoulder. In this case, we are usually stooped over, our upper chest is collapsed, and our head is no longer balanced on our neck. The neck muscles have to work hard constantly to keep the head from tipping even further forward.

"Every inch of Forward Head Posture ... can increase the weight of the head on the spine by an additional ten pounds," according to A. I. Kapandji in *The Physiology of the Joints*.[60] The head itself weighs about twelve pounds, and many of us have our head forward by two or three inches.

The man in the forward head posture photograph came to me complaining of difficulty breathing and general fatigue. His forward head posture was not the result of muscle tensions, but of flaccid trapezius muscles. As mentioned earlier, FHP often results from a dysfunction in the trapezius and sternocleidomastoid muscles; the trapezius lacks sufficient tonus, while parts of the SCM are in chronic tension. Improving the muscular tonus of these muscles, therefore, brings the head back into better alignment.

Many forms of massage and movement work well on muscles of the body generally. However, because these two muscles are innervated by cranial nerves, I use a different approach for them. The first step toward normalizing tension in either of these two muscles is doing the Basic Exercise (see Part Two). I often see that when a patient does this exercise, even for the first time, it helps bring their head back part of the way.

For further improving FHP and bringing the head back to an upright position, I also utilize two other exercises—the "Twist and Turn Exercise" and the "Salamander Exercises." You can find instructions for these exercises in Part Two.

SCAR TISSUE AS A CONTRIBUTOR TO FHP

Scar tissue forms after surgical operations in order to make the body stronger, in case a similar wound occurs at the same place in the future. The patient may know intellectually that this extra scaffolding is not necessary, because there is not likely to be another incision at the same exact place, but the connective tissue has no way of knowing this.

Although the operation itself might have been necessary or even lifesaving, the layers of muscle and fascia contract and thicken as the incision heals, and this tightening in the fascial network spreads beyond the local area of the incision to affect the entire body. Every surgical operation has this negative side effect, which is almost never addressed.

Even though there may not be much scar tissue visible on the surface, there can still be extensive buildup of scar tissue in the muscles and connective tissue under the skin, and in the deeper fascia layers. Even if the operation was done with a scope to minimize tissue damage, scars form in the deeper layers.

There should be a small amount of thick fluid between adjacent layers of muscle and connective tissue, allowing them to slide freely across one another. During an operation, however, this fluid sometimes dries out when exposed to the air so that, instead of sliding, the layers begin to stick to one another.

Also, after a surgical incision or any wound, the connective tissue cells produce extra collagen fibers that can bind one layer of muscle or fascia to an adjacent layer. When two layers have grown together, they no longer slide across each other as they once did. Many surgeons take the extra time and care to ensure that the tissues of each layer are sewn together without involving tissues from other layers.

Unfortunately, some surgeons do not understand the importance of this, and might sew layers together haphazardly in an attempt to save time and money. The result is that the muscles and connective tissue are much less flexible in that area. Scar tissue feels thicker and tougher, and it forms not just on the surface but deeper in the body. If it is from a C-section, the scar tissue goes all the way down from the surface of the skin to the uterus. If it is in the chest or abdomen, scar tissue restricts the space available for breathing.

Scarring after an operation pulls everything together into a knot; the individual layers dry out and stick together, and movement is restricted. As connective tissue on the front of the body tightens, it shortens the front of the body and pulls the head even more forward and down. Therefore, I recommend that anyone who has had chest or abdomen surgery should find a massage therapist skilled in releasing tensions from scar tissue.

The idea behind the treatment of scar tissue is to work on restrictions in each individual layer of muscle and connective tissue, and then to free the individual layers from each other so that one layer can again slide freely on the adjacent layer. I am regularly amazed by the amount of improvement that occurs in range of motion in the head and neck, flexibility in the spine, and in the posture generally after releasing scar tissue.

FHP AND SUBOCCIPITAL MUSCLE TENSION

Whereas the sternocleidomastoid and trapezius muscles provide gross rotational movements of the head on the neck, the fine-tuning of these movements comes from the small suboccipital muscles between the occiput and the first two vertebrae of the neck. Three of these muscles define an area called the suboccipital triangle. (See "Suboccipital muscles" in the Appendix.)

When these suboccipital muscles are tight, they can put pressure on the suboccipital nerve (see "Suboccipital nerve" in the Appendix) and the nearby vertebral arteries, which are embedded in the connective tissue of the suboccipital triangle. This reduces blood supply to the brainstem as well as to the five cranial nerves whose function is necessary for social engagement.

With a forward head posture, the muscles of the suboccipital triangle tighten in order to keep the chin from falling forward onto the chest. If these muscles are kept in a state of constant contraction (over months or years), they contract more and more, which further accentuates the forward head posture, and this can further reduce blood flow to the brainstem.

It is not surprising that so many people with FHP complain of headaches at the back of the neck, just under the base of the cranium, where these suboccipital muscles are located. Pressure on the suboccipital nerves often expresses itself as pain at the back of the neck. It is interesting that some clients with headaches complain that they feel as if they are not getting enough energy (blood circulation) up to their head.

I have observed that patients with asthma have poor ventral vagal function. Also, they almost always have a forward head posture. They have a stiff upper thoracic spine, and reduced lateral expansion of their chest when breathing in. Reducing FHP improves their breathing.

The Basic Exercise usually releases the tension in the suboccipital muscles. C1 rotates back into place, pressure on the vertebral arteries is reduced, the blood flow to the brainstem increases, and this in turn improves our capacity for social engagement.

Relieving Migraine Headaches

Unlike "cold lungs" (COPD), migraines do not take years off our life expectancy, but they certainly reduce the quality of our life. There are many affordable medicines for migraines, but these do not work all of the time for everyone. Some medicines are also expensive, and most have possible side effects. So many people would prefer to be free from taking medicine altogether.

Of the forty-five million people in the United States who suffer from headaches every year, twenty-eight million suffer from migraines.[61] Aside from affecting quality of life, migraine headaches are one of the most costly health problems in terms of time lost from work. This cost in the United States alone was estimated to be $17 billion a year in 2005.[62]

Migraine is Greek for "one side of the head." If the pain is not localized on one side of the head, I do not consider it a migraine. Migraine headaches, often called tension headaches, range from moderate to severe, and are usually intense, sometimes throbbing, and typically last from two hours to three days. They often occur with symptoms of autonomic dysfunction. They start suddenly and often disappear just as suddenly; this sets a migraine apart from other headaches that are sometimes described as "dull," "on both sides of the head," or "like a tight helmet," or that come on slowly, increase in intensity, and end gradually.

Migraines may be accompanied by other symptoms such as blurred vision, nausea, vomiting, fatigue, and oversensitivity to light, sound, smell, and being touched. Other accompanying symptoms can include visual distortions (seeing auras) and dizziness. Women might report that their headaches come at a specific point in their monthly cycle.

Doctors often classify migraines into different types depending on these accompanying symptoms, and patients usually want to give me detailed information about these symptoms, including how long ago the headaches started and how long they last. Although this information is important to my client, it does not help me as a therapist to treat them—I know that if I can cure their migraines, the accompanying symptoms will also disappear. To effectively treat a migraine, I need only know on which side of the head the pain appears, and which parts of the two major neck muscles are involved.

To establish this, I show clients four drawings of trigger points for the trapezius and sternocleidomastoid muscles. (These drawings are based on the work of Janet Travell, MD, and David Simons, MD, described below.) The red areas in the drawings illustrate the patterns of pain that can come from tensions in these muscles. I ask the migraine sufferer to pick out which drawing best fits the headache, and to show me exactly where she feels pain.

Without hesitating, all have been able to identify which of these four drawings best illustrates the pattern of their pain. With this information, I know exactly which muscle is involved. I am primarily interested in the *pattern of the pain,* which tells me exactly where I should intervene with my hands to bring about lasting relief. In the "Headache" drawings in the Appendix, you can find the different patterns of tension causing these headaches, the different patterns of pain, and where to massage specifically for each pattern. My discovery of this alternative approach to treating migraine headaches did not come all at once in one great epiphany, but in the form of many insights over the years. In my work with Rolfing and other forms of body-oriented therapies, most of my clients came to me because they had pain somewhere in their body.

From books by Dr. Janet Graeme Travell (1901–1997) I learned about using trigger points to successfully bring about relaxation of muscles and to relieve pain. Dr. Travell co-authored the two-volume *Myofascial Pain and Dysfunction: The Trigger Point Manual* with David G. Simons, MD, and Lois Simons[63] and served as a physician in the White House, first to John F. Kennedy and then to Lyndon Johnson.

President Kennedy had severe back pain stemming from wounds suffered when he served in the Navy in World War II. His fifth and final surgical procedure in September 1957 left him disenchanted with surgical solutions for his back pain. Later, a conservative program, including diluted salt-water injections at trigger points, provided modest relief. He wore a back brace and took hot baths several times a day, often using crutches while walking, except when he was in public view. Janet Travell, however, was able to relieve his severe and chronic back pain.

Dr. Travell's research demonstrated that tension in individual muscles generates specific patterns of pain. Most inexperienced massage therapists simply massage where it hurts, but muscle tension often produces pain and other symptoms in other parts of the body. Pain at a distance from the source of tension is called "referred pain." Dr. Travell found that treating specific points in muscles not only relieves pains near those points but can diminish referred pains as well; she called these "trigger points."

All muscles have trigger points. The therapist will often observe that they feel a little harder compared with other areas on the surface of the muscle; the patient will also feel that those points are painful. Massaging these trigger points relieves the pain in the area locally, and also relieves referred pain occurring at a distance from the tense muscle. Relieving tension in the trapezius and sternocleidomastoid muscles of the neck, by pressing the appropriate trigger points, relieves migraine headaches.

I bought two wall posters for my clinic that illustrate the trigger points of many major muscles in an easy-to-use format. Each drawing showed the pattern of pain in a muscle, the muscle involved, and where to massage that muscle in order to release the pain. When people came for pain treatment, I would ask them to point to the drawing in the posters that matched the pattern of pain they felt in their body; then I knew which muscle was involved, and which trigger points, marked with X's, I should massage to bring relief.

When I treated the trigger points on the muscles involved in migraines headaches, they disappeared even if they had bothered the clients for twenty or more years.

My clients were often amazed at how quickly I figured out where to treat them, and how effectively I could treat pains that other therapists had not been able to handle. I gave photocopies of the drawings of those muscles to my clients. In case the pain came back, they could treat themselves, or show it to another therapist treating them. About a third of the people who suffer from migraines can feel when one is about to unleash its fury. This gives them a chance to lie down, take a pill or, better yet, to use the exercises and massage described later in this section.

My next important discovery leading to a successful protocol for treating migraines derived from my experiences with biomechanical craniosacral therapy. The twelve cranial nerves exchange information between the brainstem and various parts of the body, primarily to and from regions of the head and neck. One of these nerves, CN XI or the accessory nerve, modulates tension in the sternocleidomastoid and trapezius muscles in the neck, which can cause one of several patterns of pain corresponding to the pains of migraine headaches.

Biomechanical craniosacral therapy offers specific techniques to free blockages to the eleventh cranial nerve at the point where it exits the cranium. I get the best results treating migraines when I improve the function of CN XI before releasing tension in the muscles with a light pressure on trigger points. Migraine relief is then faster and longer lasting. Most of my clients are surprised to feel relief on the very first treatment.

If the eleventh cranial nerve is not functioning properly, the ventral branch of the vagus nerve and the ninth cranial nerve are usually dysfunctional as well. Treating one of the three nerves immediately improves the function of the other two so that, in practice, we do not have to treat each of the three nerves one at a time. The Basic Exercise usually makes all three of these nerves functional.

Some writers on the subject of migraines believe that "the underlying causes of migraines are unknown"[64]—and not knowing their cause makes them hard to treat. Other studies show that a number of psychological conditions may be associated with migraines, including activity of the dorsal branch of the vagus nerve, anxiety, and bipolar disorder.[65] I find this of interest from the point of view of the Polyvagal Theory. In Chapter 6, we will look at a few psychological conditions, and note that they have a physiological aspect and are expressions of non-ventral vagal states.

Do migraines have a musculoskeletal component? Although some physiotherapists and body therapists are aware of it, the muscular component underlying migraine headaches is generally not recognized by physicians and medical researchers. *Myofascial Pain and Dysfunction: The Trigger Point Manual* shows patterns of pain on one side of the head that are caused by tension in the trapezius and the sternocleidomastoid muscles; these are the patterns I show to my clients who complain of migraine headaches, and with these they can easily identify their headache pattern.

I have found over the years that improving the function of CN X and XI, followed by releasing tension in these muscles using the appropriate trigger points, usually effectively relieves migraine headaches in a matter of minutes. I have even had success with some people who had migraines their entire life, as far back as they could remember.

In my clinic, I like to teach clients how to do the techniques themselves in the event that they are plagued by another migraine headache. Doing the Basic Exercise, they can first establish proper function in their CN X and XI. Then they can find and release the appropriate trigger points. This treatment requires no pharmaceuticals, has no side effects—and no cost.

From my successful experience treating migraines, I believe that most migraine sufferers can successfully treat themselves with the Basic Exercise and the self-help massage techniques for migraine described in Part Two, rather than taking painkillers or subjecting themselves to other conventional treatments.

In my clinic I occasionally get patients who have had migraines for many years and have tried everything else before coming to me. Perhaps they have treated their migraines with over-the-counter and/or prescription painkillers, antidepressants, beta-blockers, or drugs developed to treat epilepsy. One of the most common side effects of these drugs is liver damage, which in the worst case can eventually lead to buildup of fluids around the brain.

These clients often tell me that they take a lot of medication and would like to cut down. I remember a forty-two-year-old carpenter who was taking fifteen to twenty over-the-counter painkillers a day and was worried about negative side effects, since the directions on the bottle said to take a maximum of eight tablets a day. My client started taking his first pain-killer in the morning as soon as he opened his eyes, regardless of whether he had a headache or not. He said that he took the pills as a preventive measure so that he did not have to wait for them to take effect in case he got a migraine. He also, however, complained that the painkillers did not always work for him.

First I showed him how to treat himself with the Basic Exercise (see Part Two), which is safe, easy to learn, and easy to do. Then I showed him the four drawings of the patterns of pain that are present in most migraine headaches. When he identified the drawing that fit the pattern he was experiencing, I knew which muscles needed to relax, and which trigger points in his neck would relax the tension.

His first session with me substantially reduced the number of his head-aches and decreased the intensity of the few that did occur. If the pain returns after I give a treatment, I tell people that they can simply treat themselves as described above.

MIGRAINES: A CASE STUDY

A woman who had been suffering from migraine headaches for almost ten years came to me for treatments. She was experiencing a migraine at the time she came into my office.

On average she had one severe attack every month that usually lasted three to four days. She tried taking painkillers, but they did not help. She tried in general to avoid known migraine triggers such as heavy red wine, strong scents, bright sunshine, etc., but the migraines kept recurring. When she felt a migraine coming on, if she could withdraw and stay in bed, the attack was usually not so bad.

This woman is a journalist who wrote articles about beauty for maga-zines. She could schedule around her deadlines if she got a headache because she was working from home; she could take a day or two off, and work when she felt up to it. However, the headaches did keep her from attending many social events and enjoying her weekends off.

About a year before she came to me, this woman had started a new career as a TV journalist, which meant that she now had a harder time scheduling around her migraines. She had to show up for work and follow the shooting schedule whether or not she had a migraine, so she felt she needed a more effective treatment.

First I tested her ventral vagus (see Chapter 4) and noted that it was not functioning as it should. Then I instructed her to do the Basic Exercise, and she did this herself; I did not even need to touch her. I tested her again and saw that her ventral vagus nerve was now functioning as it should.

Then I showed her the four drawings of migraine pain patterns, and she pointed to the drawing that matched her pattern. I taught her how to use her own hands to treat the trigger points illustrated in that drawing.

I certainly could have used my hands for this treatment, but I wanted her to do it herself so that, if she experienced migraines in the future, she could come back to her own muscle memory of how to achieve positive results on her own. Although it is nice when people come back to me because they remember that I helped them in the past, I think it is better for them to help themselves rather than depending on me or any other therapist.

I asked this woman to explore the areas in her neck that generally corresponded to the location of the X's in the drawings. She used her fingers to search for areas of the muscles that were hard or painful. If an X area was not hard or painful, she just ignored it. Then I had her rub the hard or painful areas gently until she felt them relax or soften, or until the pain diminished. Although I coached her about what to do and where to put her hands, she treated herself with her own hands. By the end of the session, her migraine had disappeared.

She was able to live without migraine headaches for four and a half months. Then, when she did feel a migraine about to start, she again did the Basic Exercise and massaged the trigger points. The symptoms passed quickly and did not develop into a full-blown migraine.

CHAPTER 6

Somatopsychological Problems

A few decades ago, medical doctors began diagnosing some health problems as "psychosomatic" (meaning that the mind causes problems in the body). However, few psychiatrists and psychologists have investigated the reverse of this: is there such a thing as a somatopsychological problem, where physiology is seen to affect the mind?

The word *psychology* is derived from ancient Greek and means "study of the mind." Today, defining a problem as "psychological" usually means that a psychologist or psychiatrist first looks for the solution in the mind or emotions of their clients, most often using a verbal approach to therapy.

In this traditional, older definition, there was no mention of the body. When Freud started psychoanalysis to help people with their psychological issues, his treatment modality was 100 percent verbal. He let people talk without interruption, and he appeared to be listening. There was no dialogue; he did not even make eye contact or look at his patients face-to-face. People stayed in psychoanalysis for years, often going to sessions several times a week.

Before being trained as a psychiatrist, someone must be a medical doctor. Then they undergo their own process of psychoanalysis, which may take several years. At one point there were very few trained psychiatrists, and most people could not afford their treatment.

Psychologists created a new framework that differed from that of classical psychoanalysis. Clinical psychologists are educated over a period of just a few years in a university program. To help their patients improve their emotional states and change their behaviors, they rely on various models of the human psyche, and they enter into a dialogue with their patients using various verbal approaches. They are generally looking for solutions to specific problems. Although not as expensive as years of psychoanalysis, psychological treatment is still costly, requiring the time of a trained professional in a one-on-one situation.

Some therapists offer group therapy, which is even less expensive, since many patients share the cost of a session. However, that process is more random, since everyone in the group, trained or untrained, gives input into a session.

Today we are increasingly moving away from these modalities and relying primarily on prescription drugs to change our behaviors and emotional states. After an initial period of professional consultation to select the medicine and dosage, patients can go for long periods of time just taking their pills without needing to visit a health professional. In spite of the fact that prescription drugs can be expensive, they are cost-efficient when compared to ongoing, one-on-one therapeutic processes with psychologists or psychiatrists. However, because more and more people are taking these medications, this type of treatment means a growing expense for the individual as well as for insurance companies and the national economy.

Because psychiatry and psychology started out with an emphasis exclusively on the mind, and because of the current availability and widespread use of prescription medicines, we might be missing out on something else that can help with the health issues that these kinds of treatments intend to address. Perhaps there is something at our fingertips that has no cost or negative side effects.

In this chapter, we will look to the body to seek alternative and complementary solutions to psychological and mental health issues. We will investigate the possibility of regulating our own nervous systems and our own emotional states and behaviors. We will explore how self-help exercises and hands-on techniques can be perfectly safe and effective in achieving positive changes.

Based on my clinical experiences over the last twelve years, I believe that with a working understanding of the Polyvagal Theory many of us can help ourselves by directly treating our own autonomic nervous systems. We may be able to overcome what have been previously considered to be even intractable psychological and psychiatric issues.

EMOTIONS AND THE AUTONOMIC NERVOUS SYSTEM

Are we open, friendly, communicative, and cooperative? Are we shut down, depressed, or apathetic? Or are we angry, aggressive, anxious, fearful, or withdrawn? How do we react to other people when we are in these different states?

The way other people respond to us is based on a combination of the state they are in and the state we are in. Our emotions play out in the interaction between the state of our autonomic nervous system and theirs.

As mammals, we are social animals, and we need others. We all face challenges and uncertainty from time to time, and in order to improve our chances for survival and fulfillment we are dependent on our interaction with others—family, friends, neighbors, workmates, and our social network. How we feel in a given situation or about a specific person is a factor in our behavior. Does someone need our help? Do we enjoy sharing time with her? Is she usually supportive? Are we willing to support her? Do we work well together? Do we feel safe? Is there a chance for cooperation, sharing, and friendship?

If we are single and dating someone, is there a chance for intimacy and long-term bonding with the other person as a potential partner? If we are married or in an ongoing relationship, do we have enough time together when we are both socially engaged? The more good times we share, the more we have to draw on when the going gets tough.

Proper function of the five social-engagement cranial nerves is central to our communication and to bonding with others. These five nerves facilitate our hearing, shape the sounds of our speech, and help us to understand what other people are saying. Can we look at the other person calmly and directly, or do we shut them out of our field of vision? If we feel happy and safe, we will generally be able to carry on a normal two-way conversation, listen to what is being said, and look at the other person to exchange meaningful visual cues.

I consider the autonomic nervous system and emotional states as two sides of the same coin. If we want to improve our emotional state in order to help ourselves or others, we can accomplish this with physical actions that improve the state of our autonomic nervous system and move us out of a dorsal vagal or stress state into social engagement.

A SELF-REGULATING AUTONOMIC NERVOUS SYSTEM

Social interaction with people who are in a state of balance and social engagement is perhaps the most natural and helpful way to achieve self-regulation. If we experience a problem, it is often enough to simply talk about it with a friend. We might sit down and eat a meal, or enjoy a cup of coffee or a beer together. We might sing, dance, or go for a walk together.

Another way to self-regulate our autonomic nervous system is to do the exercises in this book. A host of other practices from cultures and traditions around the world have been used for centuries with good effect: meditation, tai chi, and yogic breathing *(pranayama),* to name a few. When we meditate, we sit still, overcoming any impulse to fight or run. We also learn to keep awake, avoiding the tendency to withdraw and dissociate. When we do tai chi, we move slowly, simulating the movements of a very relaxed state. Moving slowly also makes it easier to sense our body and to be present in it.

If we can maintain a ventral vagal state, or at least return to it quickly after stress or emotional withdrawal, we can achieve optimal health and well-being. We can open the way to realizing our human potential, enjoying being with other people, and doing what we want with our lives.

A FRESH LOOK AT COMMON PSYCHOLOGICAL DIAGNOSES

I am neither a psychologist nor a psychiatrist; however, in forty-five years as a body therapist, I have encountered many clients diagnosed by a psychologist or psychiatrist. I have also taken many courses in these areas. But I have learned the most from my clients who shared their case stories with me.

In this chapter I will present some of these stories. The stories and my commentary are purely anecdotal, based on my own experiences from my practice over the years, seen in the light of my personal and limited understanding of the Polyvagal Theory and its implications. I hope to inspire you—or perhaps provoke you—to take a fresh look at some of these issues, whether you are a trained health care professional, a consumer using health care professionals, or just someone trying to get a better understanding of your own issues in order to help yourself and/or loved ones.

I believe that there is an interrelationship between the mind, body, and emotions. Issues as different as post-traumatic stress, anxiety, phobias, and autism spectrum disorders have a somatic component, and almost all cases of so-called psychological problems include a lack of flexibility and resilience in the autonomic nervous system.

I have found it both interesting and efficacious to consider the somatic component of what we generally term "psychological issues." A great deal of healing potential becomes available when we consider the possibility of identifying and treating the physical manifestations of the autonomic nervous system at the outset of psychiatric and psychological treatments.

If there is indeed a unity of mind-body-emotion, it follows that we might be able to help people with psychological diagnoses by starting their treatment with body-therapy techniques, especially if these can bring them out of a state of chronic stress or dorsal vagal activity and toward greater flexibility of autonomic response.

Anxiety and Panic Attacks

Since the beginnings of psychiatry at the end of the nineteenth century, there has been a strong focus on anxiety disorders.

Occasional anxiety is a normal part of life. We might feel anxious when faced with a problem at work, before taking a test, or when making an important decision. But anxiety disorders involve more than temporary worry or fear. For some of us, anxiety can become excessive, and while we may realize this, we may have difficulty controlling it, so that anxiety may negatively affect our day-to-day living.

For a person with an anxiety disorder, the anxiety does not go away and can get worse over time. The feelings can interfere with daily activities, such as job performance, schoolwork, and relationships. Modern surveys find that some form of anxiety disorder affects as many as 18 percent of people in the United States in a typical twelve-month period; over the course of their lifetimes, 30 percent will experience some anxiety disorder.[66]

What we call "fear" is a psychological process involving nervous-system activation in the face of a threatening situation. Fear can immobilize us (via dorsal vagal activity) or mobilize us to fight or flight (from activity of the sympathetic chain). Physical symptoms can include rapid heartbeat (tachycardia), increased respiration, the release of high levels of stress hormones, blushing, difficulty speaking, and sweating in the palms of the hands, soles of the feet, and armpits.

Anxiety is similar to fear in terms of its physical manifestations. However, anxiety may not necessarily occur in response to an actual situation. Something can remind us of an event in our past, or we may project our imagination onto something that might happen in the future. In either case, the threat is not happening now. Nonetheless, this emotional state is real, and it exists in the body in present time.

When anxious, we find that we cannot get the concerns out of our minds. If another person tells us there is nothing to worry about, it does not quiet our minds; it can sometimes upset us even more. We may respond, "Are you saying my feelings aren't real?"

Panic attacks are brief experiences of intense terror and apprehension. They arise abruptly and usually peak in less than ten minutes, although uncomfortable feelings can continue for several hours. Sometimes the specific cause of a panic attack is not apparent. In other cases, we can ascertain that it was triggered by general factors such as stress, fear, or even excessive exercise.

People having a panic attack display recognizable signs of fear. Their physical symptoms include trembling, shaking, confusion, dizziness, nausea, and difficulty breathing. Their appearance looks strained, their skin is pale, and they have increased sweating in the palms of their hands, soles of their feet, and armpits. Their sweat has a characteristic odor.

Dogs and other mammals respond immediately to body smells arising from different emotional states. People also react instinctively to the smell of fear in another person, even though they might not be conscious of it. Many people try to mask olfactory signs of fear and anxiety by using perfumes, deodorants, or foot powders. However, it is difficult to mask a cold, clammy hand and a limp handshake when meeting someone.

Sometimes anxiety and panic attacks can be effectively addressed with exercises or hands-on techniques that help bring us out of a state of sympathetic nervous system or dorsal vagal activation into a state of social engagement.

We sometimes refer to "the drop that made the pitcher overflow." If an anxious person uses the Basic Exercise regularly, they can minimize the frequency and intensity of panic or anxiety attacks and, in some cases, even prevent attacks. Doing the exercise regularly is like reducing the amount of water in the pitcher, so that it can hold many more drops without overflowing.

It is also important to be aware that anxiety can be a side effect of a prescription drug, or indicate a substance-abuse problem, since medications and other drugs alter the state of the autonomic nervous system.

CASE STUDY: ANXIETY AND PANIC ATTACKS

I had a client who was bothered by anxiety and panic attacks that were keeping her from acting on her desire to have a baby. She also experienced pain in the right side of her abdomen.

The anxiety had started fifteen years earlier, when she was eighteen years old and had a surgical operation to remove her ileocecal valve. Problems with the ileocecal valve can be debilitating, and often occur with colitis, abdominal pain, groin pain, bloating, unpleasant body odor, gas, distension of the belly, and breathing problems such as asthma and "cold lungs."

The ileocecal valve controls the flow of chyme from the small intestine into the large intestine. Chyme is the thick, semifluid mass of partly digested food and secretions formed in the stomach and small intestine during digestion. Normally, the ileocecal valve is closed most of the time, only opening for short periods to allow the passage of chyme. When the chyme reaches the large intestine, excess water is absorbed into the body, and the remaining fiber and other wastes are packed together, formed into feces, and eliminated.

Problems arise if the ileocecal valve does not open properly. Problems also occur if it stays open too long, allowing chyme from the small intestine to move unrestricted into the large intestine, or to move backwards from the large into the small intestine.

In addition to anxiety symptoms, this client had occasional short periods of intense pain on the right side of her abdomen (where the ileocecal valve is located or, in her case, had been located before her surgery). Her doctor took her physical pains quite seriously and wanted to be sure that the operation had gone properly. They did several MRIs and two laparoscopic explorations, but found that everything looked all right; they could find nothing to explain her pain.

When I asked why she had had the operation in the first place, she said that it was because of pain. But years after the operation, she still had pain in the same area. And despite her psychological pain and suffering, the surgeon expressed no interest in her symptoms of anxiety, even though these had appeared shortly after the operation. Also, no doctor had ever evaluated the function of her autonomic nervous system.

The dorsal branch of the vagus nerve innervates most of the organs of digestion, including the small intestine, the ileocecal valve, and the ascending and transverse parts of the large intestine. It receives sensory input from the organs themselves, and exerts motor control over their functions.

The first thing that I did in my treatment was to evaluate the state of her nervous system by looking at the back of her throat when she said, "ah-ah-ah." The uvula pulled to one side (indicating dysfunction of the pharyngeal branch of the ventral vagus nerve, described in Chapter 4). I also did the Trap Squeeze Test (see Chapter 5) to check the level of tension in the two sides of her trapezius muscles. There was a clear difference between her right and left sides.

My first objective was to help get the woman's autonomic nervous system into a ventral vagal state. I instructed her on how to do the Basic

Exercise. One of the great things about this exercise is that clients can do it themselves. It took less than two minutes for me to teach her how to do the Basic Exercise, and less than two minutes for her to do it. After she did the exercise, she felt much better, and she reported that she no longer felt anxious.

The muscular tension in her trapezius on the tense side had also relaxed; when I squeezed the trapezius muscles, the muscular tension was similar on both sides. To make doubly sure that there had been a desirable change, I looked at the back of her throat and saw her uvula lifting symmetrical on both sides.

I also performed an osteopathic visceral-massage technique to relax tensions in the ileocecal valve, which usually eliminates pain immediately.

This client's surgeon assumed that the operation was a success, in terms of its limited objective of removing her ileocecal valve. Until she consulted me, however, no one considered the possibility that her operation had been a traumatic experience that left her autonomic nervous system in a state of dorsal vagal activity.

With appropriate treatment, this client made the transition out of a debilitating state of anxiety and into the desirable state of social engagement. I emphasized to her that she had made the positive change all by herself, and told her that she could always do the exercise in the future if she ever felt anxiety again.

Then I asked her to think about the difficulties triggered by her anxiety in the past. Just thinking about my question was enough to put her into a tailspin, into another state of anxiety. She lost her smile and held her breath, and the skin on her face went pale. So I asked her to repeat the Basic Exercise, and she again told me that she felt better. She looked more relaxed, with good color in her face, and her breathing was deeper. She also told me that she felt the change from anxiety to calm.

When I asked her once again to think about the trouble that the anxiety had caused her, she was able to remain calm, and said she thought she could manage the anxiety on her own in the future. I tested her autonomic nervous system again and found that she was still in a state of ventral vagal activity. She felt no pain.

These improvements came in a single session. The client thought it was a miracle, after all the pain and anxiety that she had suffered before her treatment with me. For me, although I was flattered to hear this, it seemed a shame that the surgeon never examined her autonomic nervous system and did not have a knowledge of visceral massage.

A year and a half later, I received an email from this woman. She thanked me for my treatment and wrote that she no longer suffered from anxiety. I suggested that she come for another session with me in order to release any tension that might still remain in the scar tissue, since her long-term improvement depended not only on improving the function of the vagus nerve but on release of the trauma held in scar tissue locally.

Pain in the body can cause anxiety. A surgical operation, even though it was consciously chosen, is still an assault on the integrity of the body and, like any trauma, can leave its mark.

SOCIAL REGULATION OF ANXIETY STATES

Simple, everyday social interactions with supportive family, friends, and colleagues can help regulate our psychological state. We should not underestimate the importance of chatting, small talk, and simple social situations like eating together, having a cup of coffee, or taking a walk with someone. Good social relationships help our nervous systems to self-regulate.

Like weeding a garden, if we have been victimized we should eliminate or minimize contact with people who make us feel bad, and maximize the time spent with people who support us and leave us feeling better.

When we have been traumatized and then become socially engaged and leave treatment, we will encounter new situations in which we might again feel threatened. At first we may need a therapist's support to be restored to a state of social engagement, but the ideal outcome is having the tools to be able to reach it ourselves. Each time we get back up, we weaken the hold that the traumatic pattern has had on us; we can rest and restore ourselves, making more energy available for us to meet the next challenges in life.

If we feel that our social network is inadequate, we may also experience helpful and positive interactions by turning to health professionals such as massage therapists, counselors, coaches, psychologists, or psychiatrists. We may choose to consult a religious or spiritual teacher or leader. We may also find solace in prayer, or read religious and spiritual texts to help put things in perspective.

TREATING ANXIETY IN CHILDREN

Parents or other adults often tell children, "There is nothing to be afraid of." In many cases, this reassurance from a loving parent or a trusted close friend is enough to make someone feel safe.

It would be even more effective, however, if the adult began by saying, "I understand that you are feeling afraid." This gives the child assurance that they have been heard, and the knowledge that fear (like other emotions) is a normal life experience.

The adult can then continue: "There is nothing to be afraid of. It will be all right." Then a little hug helps, so that the child gets positive physical contact and can feel the relaxation of the adult.

Phobias

Phobias are the single largest category of anxiety disorders, and they can be incapacitating. A phobia is characterized by an experience of extreme fear, with a specific trigger that sets off a state of anxiety or a panic attack. Physiologically, fear arises from a reaction in the sympathetic division of the autonomic nervous system.

Between 5 and 12 percent of the world's entire population is estimated to suffer from phobic disorders.[67] Sufferers typically anticipate terrifying consequences from encountering the object of their fear. They want to flee, but they are immobilized. They may understand intellectually that their reaction of fear is irrational and out of proportion to the potential danger, but they are still overwhelmed by their fear.[68]

Psychologists and therapists often focus on the object of fear, such as heights (acrophobia), not having enough space (claustrophobia), or spiders (arachnophobia). Their diagnoses focus on the triggers, which may or may not be easily linked to specific biographical events. A phobia might be caused by experiences from the past—for example, when someone encountered a threatening person or a life-threatening situation. A phobia can just as easily come from a virtual experience, in which the person suffering the phobia did not actually experience the event—for example, it might have come from someone else telling a story, or from watching a scene in a movie.

A list of phobias in Wikipedia—which notes that this list is incomplete and invites readers to add to it—included twenty-three entries that begin with the letter *A* alone. This gives us an idea of how wide-ranging this problem is, and gives the impression that almost anything can trigger the same kind of anxiety response.

In order to better understand something, we tend to classify it and give it a name. But rather than considering ablutophobia (fear of washing) as basically different from acousticophobia (fear of noise), for example, it may be more useful to move our focus away from the triggers and toward an understanding of the physiological activity in the autonomic nervous system in all cases of phobia.

You might be able to assist people with phobias if you can help them return from a state of extreme fear to a state of social engagement using the Basic Exercise (see Part Two). The effect can be similar to what parents do when they help their children by hugging and holding them until the child relaxes and feels safe again.

Whereas physical contact is natural between a parent and a child, in a professional psychological intervention there should be no physical contact. Therefore, a therapist needs to find another way to make the client feel safe again, and directing a client to use the Basic Exercise might be an ideal solution.

Antisocial Behavior and Domestic Violence

Most people consider normal human behavior as an expression of positive social values. When people are not socially engaged, however, it is often hard for others to understand their behavior.

Some people who commit aggressive acts do not have any idea that there is anything wrong with them; they are convinced that the other person caused or justifies their behavior. In other words, aggressive people believe their actions to be a natural response: "He had it coming." They might even consider their action as helping the other person: "It's the only way that she will learn."

It may be difficult to understand why seemingly normal people commit violent crimes. Observing their actions, we can conclude that they lack empathy, but that does not tell us what is going on inside them. What drives them? Is it territory, power, money, sex, jealousy, or maybe alienation? Or is it just an unpleasant feeling that intensifies and then explodes like a bomb into antisocial behavior? Many violent crimes are not premeditated.

I heard an ex-convict in Denmark speak in a radio interview. He had been in prison for most of his adult years for many different offenses, including several bank robberies. After leaving prison, he joined a voluntary rehabilitation program that included yoga, meditation, and breathing exercises, and felt that this program had given him control over his emotions and his actions.

When the moderator asked him if he had any remorse about the effects of his actions on his victims, he said no—not when he was committing the crimes. "In a war," he said, "the enemy soldiers have no faces." It wasn't until he had stopped his criminal activities and had been in the rehabilitation program that he started to think of the effects on the other people.

The perpetrator of a violent crime may or may not have a rational motive that other people can understand, but still somehow they entered a psychophysiological state of fight or flight that drove their actions.

"NICE GUY" COMMITS WAR CRIMES

A young man enlisted in the army to serve his country, and was trained to fight. He also learned the rules of conduct expected for soldierly behavior in a war zone, according to the Geneva Convention—not to torture, not to kill civilians, not to rape, not to steal.

Almost all soldiers adhere to these rules, but occasionally something else happens. On a routine patrol, this young soldier's best friend was killed by an enemy sniper. Then a few more of his friends were killed or wounded in an ambush by a roadside bomb. Suddenly, the soldier snapped. He ran amok, gathered a few innocent civilians, tied them up, raped one of the women in front of her family, and then massacred them all. He was brought to trial by the army, found guilty, and sentenced to a long prison term.

The soldier's parents and friends back home were shocked. They could not believe that he was capable of doing anything like this: "He was such a nice boy, and he came from a good family." "This was so unlike him." "He had always been positive, helpful, and friendly when he was growing up." The term "intermittent explosive disorder" describes the occurrence of discrete episodes of aggression to other people or to property. The individual may say that the explosive behavior was preceded by a sense of tension or arousal. From the perspective of the autonomic nervous system, intermittent explosive behavior is an example of extreme mobilization with fear. Like anxiety, it results in uncontrollable fight or flight behavior.

Individual acts of intermittent explosive behavior show up regularly on the evening news—shooting children and teachers at an elementary school, blowing up a church, or suicide bombings. We watch the reports, we are fascinated by the events, and we think to ourselves that we cannot understand how someone could do something like that to other people.

The individual's behavior does not seem justified; the violent episodes appear to be grossly out of proportion to any provocation. If you ask the person why they committed the act, they may not be able to give an answer or, if they do, it will not make sense to anyone else. They might say that they felt a sense of relief immediately afterward. However, feelings of relief are usually short lived, and when the level of tension rises again, subsequent episodes can follow.

CASE STUDY: ONGOING DOMESTIC VIOLENCE

Domestic violence is quite different than facing the enemy in a war, or being the victim of random violence in the street. Some people become victims of domestic violence simply when a love relationship goes sour.

Let's shift our focus from the perpetrator of violence to the victim. A man and woman are attracted to each other, and they spend more time together; they eventually move in together and start a family. She feels safe with him; she might even feel that he is her protector. Then one day, he suddenly loses his temper and hits her. She is surprised and shocked, and starts to cry.

When things settle down, he gives her a hug and says he is sorry. She asks him to promise that he will never do it again, and he promises. After a while, they put the incident behind them. At first she is wary, but he seems to have settled down. Their life together goes on as before—almost.

One day, out of the blue, he gets angry and hits her again. She is not only in physical pain, she also feels threatened. When his anger fades, he says he regrets it. Again, they kiss and make up, but as this cycle repeats itself, at some point she moves from feeling safe to living in constant fear. He is physically stronger, so she cannot win in a physical fight. She sometimes fantasizes about hitting him with a frying pan while he sleeps.

She considers taking the children and running away. But where would she go? Where would she live? How could she support herself and her children? What would other people say? She feels trapped, and cannot see any viable choices. Reluctantly, she stays. But the joy that she originally felt from being with him at the start of their relationship is dead. He notices that she has cooled to him emotionally, which upsets him even further: "What is wrong with you?"

After a few more incidents, she loses any will to fight back or run away. She just endures, and dissociates from her body when she is attacked, as if she does not care what is happening to her. She may even see herself from a distance when she is being hit. She is just hoping that this will soon be over. But eventually, she even stops hoping.

This woman has made a long, unwanted journey from love (social engagement) to mobilization with fear (fighting back and/or running away) to immobilization with fear. She has succumbed to a state that we can describe as "freeze," with the accompanying emotions of apathy, detachment, and hopelessness. Perhaps giving in and being passive when he attacked her helped her to survive; she might have been even more injured if she had fought back, or if she ran away and he came after her.

She is too ashamed to tell other people, so she suffers alone. The responses of others may often sound like condemnation: "If it was so terrible, why didn't you run away?" "Why didn't you call me? I would have helped you." "How could you let him continue to do this to you?" "If you were so stupid and did not do anything, it's your own fault." These comments seem unfair when what she needs is a feeling of being understood, a feeling of safety and support.

Other people are unlikely to understand that her nervous system had been hammered down the evolutionary scale from social engagement to stress and finally to withdrawal and apathy. It was her traumatized nervous system that contributed to her behavior. People assumed that she was the same person they knew before—a rational, well-functioning, and socially engaged person. People can be quick to judge without understanding the instinctive, emotional mechanisms behind such changes.

As a first step, a woman who has been abused needs to find a safe environment where she is free from further abuse. The events in the past have already occurred, and we cannot change them, but we can change the way that we react to them emotionally.

Is it possible to recover from these abuses and return to a normal life? By the time that the woman I've just described came to me for her first session, she was already out of the relationship. The first thing I did was to test the function of the ventral branch of her vagus nerve. Not surprisingly, I found her in a state of dorsal vagal activity. Near the end of the first treatment, I tested her again and found that she had come up to a state of social engagement. Before ending the session, I did some additional work on her neck and back, and she told me that she felt much better.

However, when she returned for her next session two weeks later, she was back in a state of pain, confusion, withdrawal, and apathy. Again she responded positively to the session, and came back up to a level of social engagement. She returned several more times. Each time she left my office, she had come up to social engagement, and the positive effects lasted longer and longer. Over time, my treatments were enough to bring her out of fear, sadness, and despair. Every time that she got back to a state of social engagement, she was less affected by the more difficult emotional states. When a person is socially engaged even some of the time, their interaction with others can be enough to begin to regulate their own nervous system.

This client came to me before I had developed and tested the Basic Exercise. After a few sessions, I taught her how to release the tension at the back of her neck with the Neuro-Fascial Release Technique described in Part Two. Rather than needing to come to me for a session each time, she could use the technique to help regulate herself whenever she felt afraid, angry, or powerless.

DOMESTIC VIOLENCE: NOT JUST MEN BEATING WIVES

Men can be beaten by their wives, children beaten by their parents, and parents beaten by their children. Although individuals seldom talk about having been sexually victimized or physically abused, domestic violence is a more serious problem than many people realize, since most people do not readily admit to being a victim of domestic violence.

When I discuss domestic violence in front of a class, although they do not say anything, I can see strong emotional reactions in the faces of many women. They may have experienced violent behavior from a father who hit them to make a point about how they should behave, or a date who had expectations about sex that they did not fulfill, or a husband over a disagreement about the family budget. It might also be that these women were thinking about a girlfriend, daughter, mother, or someone else close to them who was a victim of domestic violence.

How widespread is the problem of domestic violence, interpersonal violence, and stalking?

The US government's Centers for Disease Control and Prevention (CDC) conducts an ongoing National Intimate Partner and Sexual Violence Survey.[69] They have found interpersonal violence, sexual violence, and stalking to be pervasive in the United States. Intimate partner violence occurs between two people in a close relationship, including current and former spouses as well as dating partners. The violence tracked included hurting or trying to hurt a partner by hitting, kicking, or other kinds of physical force. The frequency of such violence exists along a continuum from a single episode to ongoing battering.

The CDC reports the following in a report titled *Intimate Partner Violence in the United States—2010:*[70]

- Nearly one in five women (18%) and one in seventy-one men (1.4%) have been raped in their lifetime.

- One in four women (25%) and one in seven men (14%) have been the victim of "severe" physical violence by an intimate partner.

- One in six women (17%) and one in nineteen men (5%) have been stalked during their lifetime.

- Women who experienced physical violence by an intimate partner, or rape or stalking by any perpetrator, in their lifetimes were more likely than women who did not experience these to have asthma, diabetes, and irritable bowel syndrome.

- Men and women who experienced these forms of violence were more likely to report frequent headaches, chronic pain, difficulty sleeping, activity limitations, poor physical health, and poor mental health than men and women who did not experience them.

It should be noted that statistics such as these will always underestimate the problem because many victims feel ashamed or threatened, and often they do not report such violence to police or health care practitioners, or even talk about it to friends or family.

The majority of this victimization starts early in life. Often intimate-partner violence starts with emotional abuse, and can progress to physical abuse, sexual assault, or a mixture of both. The longer the violence continues, the more serious are the psychological effects.

The traumatic experiences have both short-term and long-term consequences. Symptoms may include flashbacks, panic attacks, and trouble sleeping. Victims are often left with low self-esteem, can have a hard time trusting others, and experience difficulties being in relationships. The anger, fear, withdrawal, and helplessness that victims feel may lead to eating disorders, symptoms arising from activity of the dorsal circuit of the vagus nerve, and suicidal thoughts. Intimate-partner violence is linked to harmful health behaviors when victims try to cope with their trauma in unhealthy ways such as smoking, drinking, taking drugs, or having risky sex.

When a person is being violated, their nervous system is often in a state of shock or shutdown in which they are vulnerable to hypnotic suggestions, i.e., whatever is said to them by their abuser is fully accepted without critical evaluation. Sometimes victims of abuse have also been threatened that "If you ever tell anyone about this, I will kill you."

This can make it difficult or even impossible to get a victim to talk about what happened. A therapist who suspects that this is the case can ask: "Just answer me, yes or no—has anyone ever threatened to harm you if you speak about this?" If they say "yes," the therapist may have unlocked the door, if the patient is no longer under the compulsion to refrain from talking about what happened.

BRAIN CHANGES FROM DOMESTIC VIOLENCE

With traumatized victims as well as perpetrators, there are actual changes in the structures and function of their brains, especially in the amygdala.

The amygdala lies in the temporal lobe, in the midbrain. It is involved in how we respond emotionally to events and information, and contributes to determining how we behave when faced with potential risks. On scans, the amygdala shows increased activity during negative emotional experiences, and when we endure repeated or prolonged periods of stress, our amygdala becomes enlarged. An enlarged amygdala can make it easier to go into a state of stress or shutdown.[71]

The hippocampus is in the temporal lobes next to the amygdala, and it is where we store our non-traumatic memories. As the amygdala enlarges, the hippocampus shrinks from continued exposure to threatening and dangerous experiences.[72]

MOVING OUT OF THE PAST AND RECONNECTING TO FUTURE DREAMS

If we have suffered a trauma, we will recover more quickly if we can remember our life dreams, mission, and/or goals, which give meaning to our lives.

I asked my client who had been domestically abused, "What is the dream that you had for your life, which you have forgotten? What do you want to do?" She said that she wanted to make a good life for herself and her son. In this way she began to look forward to creating her future rather than fixating on what happened in the past.

My clinical experience is that the victim of a single traumatic experience can usually return to a normal state quickly. By contrast, the victim of domestic violence may have suffered a series of assaults, both physical and psychological, over a long period of time, and is therefore less likely to bounce back quickly.

A successful treatment outcome requires lifting the patient back up to the level of social engagement again and again until they are stable enough to be self-regulating and function normally. Recovering their previous dreams is helpful in this process.

Post-Traumatic Stress Disorder (PTSD)

Post-traumatic stress disorder (PTSD), sometimes referred to as post-traumatic stress syndrome (PTSS), has become a common diagnosis. With the wars in Iraq and Afghanistan, we have become increasingly aware of the enormous number of veterans afflicted with post-traumatic stress.

TRAUMA AND THE AUTONOMIC NERVOUS SYSTEM

Ideally, if we have a resilient autonomic nervous system, we rebound to a state of social engagement after a period of time following a traumatic event. Unfortunately, many people do not bounce back.

Everyone experiences events that are intense, shocking, and distressing, but we react differently to similar events. Some of us are able to get over them quickly, return to a state of balance, equilibrium, and social engagement, and get on with our lives. Others are changed by what happened, and the effects can be long-lasting, draining, and even incapacitating. The negative consequences can even last for the rest of the person's life. If a person is locked into a state of spinal sympathetic activity, "post-traumatic stress" is an accurate description.

However, after a trauma, not everyone is left in a state of chronic stress. Many people are actually left in a state of dorsal vagal activity with depressive behavior, and describing their condition as "post-traumatic stress" is inaccurate, confusing, and leads to ineffective treatments. It would be more accurate to talk about two different outcomes after a trauma: a chronic, post-traumatic, spinal sympathetic activation state (the fight-or-flight stress response), or a post-traumatic state of chronic dorsal vagal activity (withdrawal or shutdown).

Sometimes a person with PTSD/PTSS flip-flops between these two states, both of which prevent a state of social engagement. The problem for many soldiers returning home with a diagnosis of post-traumatic stress is that often the people treating them have not found effective treatments. Sadly, many men and women who have served their country in battle therefore wind up socially isolated, and an alarmingly high number of them commit suicide.

I find that simply using the term "PTSD" is not specific enough, is misleading, and often causes confusion. The label "post-traumatic stress" describes an ongoing physical and emotional reaction to an event that happened sometime in the past. It does not indicate the nature of the problems that are currently resulting from that trauma; it just acknowledges that something traumatic occurred and that the repercussions are ongoing.

Many patients who come to my clinic with a diagnosis of post-traumatic stress are not stressed in their nervous system (via spinal sympathetic chain activation) but are actually in a chronic dorsal vagal state. They are not mobilized into fight or flight but immobilized into fear, apathy, and hopelessness. Trying to treat them as if they are stressed can therefore be confusing and counterproductive.

We get a clearer and more useful picture by differentiating between post-traumatic stress and post-traumatic shutdown. Are the patient's behaviors and symptoms a sign of sympathetic nervous system activity, or of dorsal branch activity? Sympathetic chain activity results in what we usually describe as stress behaviors, while dorsal vagal activity leaves a person withdrawn and exhibiting depressive behavior. Shutdown to any degree occurs from a surge of activity in the dorsal (old) vagus branch. Mammals share this shutdown reaction with all the other phyla and almost all vertebrates, all the way down the evolutionary ladder to fish without jaws such as lampreys.

When treating post-traumatic stress, therapists tend to focus on the trauma itself rather than the psychophysiological fixation that followed the event. Recalling the experience and telling someone else about it is certainly one way to ease post-traumatic stress, but it is not the only way, and it can often backfire, as the person can become re-traumatized by recounting it. In many cases, it is easier and more effective for a therapist to bypass recall of the event, and work with exercises or hands-on treatments to restore a state of social engagement.

A project in Denmark involved a group of therapists who treated victims of trauma from the wars in Afghanistan and Iraq. The therapists included traditional psychologists, a craniosacral therapist, and body therapists using various modalities. All of the subjects received the same number of sessions, which included both verbal and nonverbal therapies. Some started with craniosacral therapy, followed by other body therapies, and others started with more traditional, verbal forms of therapy.

Looking back on the results, the therapists noticed that the subjects who started with the nonverbal craniosacral therapy had better results than the subjects who started by talking about what they had experienced. One of the psychologists in the group, Marc Levin, speculated that when people felt safe and relaxed after the body therapy, they felt more robust and therefore more open when they started to talk about what they had experienced. By contrast, when people talked about their experiences first, it seemed harder for them to let go of it; some of them may have actually restimulated the trauma.[73]

When people recall traumatic events in a therapy session, they may go into a hypnotic trance and restimulate the emotional state from that event. If the therapist makes a comment such as, "That was terrible," the remark can be imprinted on top of the person's own experience, so that it is no longer only the client's own belief. Now there is another person—an authority figure—who agrees with the grievance, and this may reinforce its effect. It is thus possible for people to leave their session in worse shape than when they came in.

DORSAL BRANCH ACTIVITY AND PTSD

The goal of my treatments for people with a diagnosis of PTSD is to lift them out of a state of activity in their spinal sympathetic circuit or dorsal vagal nerve, and to bring them into the state of social engagement. The next challenge is to help them stay socially engaged by repeating this whenever necessary.

It's incorrect to assume that activity of the dorsal branch is a purely psy-chological issue to be treated verbally; it is more aptly termed a psy-chophysiological state. Medical doctors often treat mental manifestations of dorsal branch activity biochemically, with antidepressant medications, many of which work as stimulants and create an aroused state in the nervous system. This helps people to mobilize generally, but it does not bring about desirable social behaviors, or states of happiness or joy.

A new understanding of stress and the role of the vagus nerve branches can be a great help in treating many psychiatric and psychological disorders. Physiological states driven by activation of visceral organs through the dorsal vagal branch result in a tremendous drain of resources and loss of quality of life—not only for the individuals themselves, their families, and the people around them, but through their economic impact on society in the treatment of these psychological issues. I believe that it is possible to bring a depressed person up to the highest level of autonomic function with the simple and cost-free hands-on techniques and exercises described in this book.

RESTORING FUNCTION AFTER A TRAUMATIC EVENT

The autonomic nervous system normally has an inherent capacity to self-regulate. If we feel safe in both our environment and our body, then it is natural to be socially engaged—to share and be at ease with others. Similarly, we can be immobilized without fear in order to rest, rebuild the body, and reproduce.

Social interaction with other people where we feel safe often restores our ability to return from stress or shutdown to social engagement. However, this does not always happen. The actual situation may be over; we have stopped running or fighting, and we are now free of the threat or danger—but our nervous system can become stuck in the past, and remain in a state of fight, flight, or freeze (dissociation). Post-traumatic stress occurs when the survival responses of fight, flight, or freeze have been aroused but not fully discharged.

When our nervous system is deregulated, we dissociate. We lose contact with our body, with other people, or with the here and now. We therefore become ineffective and vulnerable. Many commonly used phrases describe this; "out of touch," "not with it," "beside myself." In terms of the nervous system, we have lost function in the ventral branch of the vagus nerve. This can be observed by the vagal-function testing described in Chapter 4.

The trick for restoring self-regulating vagal function is to do something to get ourselves grounded again, to come back to our senses, be in our body, and return to the here and now. Some of us are helped by meditation, some by prayer, others by going fishing or getting away to a quiet place alone to be able to think things through.

In Part Two of this book, I present some exercises that help most people to get back in touch with themselves again by restoring ventral vagal function within a few minutes. I also present a hands-on technique called the Neuro-Fascial Release Technique by which one person can help another to restore their vagal function.

Some of us might seek the assistance of a therapist, coach, or teacher. The important thing is not what these health care professionals call their method, or what positive results they claim they can deliver, but whether or not their methods actually work for us. If tests showed that the ventral vagus nerve was dysfunctional before the intervention, then the same tests should show that the ventral vagus nerve has become functional after the intervention is applied.

If we are trying to restore the regulation of our nervous system with social interaction, we must be sure that the people with whom we choose to interact are themselves well functioning. A simple way of evaluating this is to ask ourselves, "When I am with them, do I feel better afterward?" We have all had experiences of being with people and feeling the worse for it.

Once we are balanced and self-regulating again, we should find that we have greater resilience when we are with the same people who brought us down before. Ideally, we will be less affected by them, or at least recover more quickly. Although we can sometimes cut down on the amount of time that we spend with people who upset us, we cannot always avoid them, so it is helpful to be able to respond more resiliently.

It is also important to be patient. Helping ourselves successfully even once will make it easier the next time. Being alive entails meeting a constant succession of challenges, threats, and dangers, and regulation is an ongoing process of successfully addressing the next difficulty when it arises. We will have an easier time meeting a new challenge if we can stay grounded, do not become upset, and maintain or quickly recover a well-functioning ventral branch of the vagus nerve.

Depression and the Autonomic Nervous System

Depression continues to be the leading cause of medical disability in the United States and Canada, accounting for nearly 10 percent of all medical disability.[74] In recent years, medical doctors have been prescribing more and more antidepressants.[75] In Denmark, where I live, almost 8.3 percent of the population takes antidepressants.[76] The most common form of treatment of depression is antidepressant medications, which are currently ranked third among prescription drugs in the United States, with global sales of more than $9.8 billion in 2013.[77]

People with a diagnosis of depression, or people in a depressed state, typically lose interest in activities that once were pleasurable. They experience loss of appetite, overeating, or other digestive problems. They have reduced energy, and become inactive, introverted, apathetic, helpless, and asocial. They can feel sad, anxious, empty, hopeless, worthless, guilty, irritable, ashamed, or restless. They may experience lethargy, lack of energy, and a lack of goal-oriented activity. They can have problems concentrating, remembering details, or making decisions, and are often plagued by the aches and pains of fibromyalgia. They may contemplate, attempt, or actually commit suicide. These can all be symptoms of activity in the dorsal branch of the vagus nerve.

If we consult with a doctor because we are not feeling good, the doctor might ask questions and ascertain from our responses that we are depressed or stressed. Rather than considering the possibility that the condition is transient, the doctor assumes that it is semipermanent, and we are put on medication. Often there is a period of adjusting the dose until we feel better. We may then stay on the medicine for months or even years.

Many people who come to me wish to stop taking their medication. Although I support them in this desire, I tell them to only do so in consultation with the physician who prescribed it. Also, I recommend looking on the internet to learn about the negative side effects of the medicine, and to find out whatever information is available about withdrawal symptoms that might occur if they stop taking it.

A study published in the *Journal of the American Medical Association* showed that antidepressant prescriptions work no better than placebos in mild cases of depression.[78] It is well known that these medicines often have negative side effects. Yet antidepressants are still the most commonly consumed class of medication in the U.S., with 270 million prescriptions written for them each year.[79]

This raises some obvious questions: Why are doctors prescribing so many antidepressants? Could we benefit by taking a new approach? I believe the underlying problem is a lack of understanding of the nature of the autonomic nervous system, which should normally be flexible, resilient and only temporarily affected by stressors. The Polyvagal Theory may point the way to this new approach.

The medical literature has generally focused on the physiology of chronic stress, with less attention given to the physiology underlying depression. When people come to my clinic with a diagnosis of depression from a psychologist or psychiatrist, or when they exhibit depressive behavior, I find that that their problem is usually accompanied by a state of activity in the dorsal branch of their vagus nerve.

Prior to the Polyvagal Theory, dorsal vagal issues lacked a physiological model in terms of the nervous system, and perhaps that is why it has been so difficult to find safe, effective medicine-free treatments for conditions such as depression. Stephen Porges's Polyvagal Theory focuses on the relationships of the autonomic nervous system, the emotions, and our behavior, and his work has awakened a growing interest in applications of these understandings by psychologists, psychiatrists, and an array of gifted, insightful trauma therapists.

Bipolar Disorder

Bipolar disorder is a behavioral pattern marked by periods of heightened activity, elation, and euphoria ("mania"), alternating with periods of depressive behavior.

Mania is characterized by abnormally elevated energy levels and an elated, jubilant, euphoric mood. Periods of mania are followed by periods of activity of the dorsal branch of the vagus nerve, experienced as low energy. In some people, these mood swings are separated by periods of "normal" feelings; in other individuals, states of dorsal branch activity and mania alternate with no respite. Such people are often dissociated from sensing their body, and can suffer from psychotic symptoms such as delusions and hallucinations. Bipolar issues affect up to 4 percent of the U.S. population.[80]

From the perspective of the Polyvagal Theory, the manic phase can be seen as activation of the spinal sympathetic chain. In a manic state, the person expends great amounts of energy and takes many actions without necessarily enjoying or being satisfied by them.

In my clinic, many clients tell me that they have been given a diagnosis by a professional psychologist or psychiatrist. I am not trained or qualified to make psychological or psychiatric diagnoses; my observations are anecdotal, based on treatment of these clients. It seems remarkable that the same approach—techniques for establishing social engagement—can help so many people with different psychological or psychiatric diagnoses, including bipolar disorder.

CASE STUDY: BIPOLAR DISORDER

A few years ago, a woman in her fifties came to me for craniosacral therapy. I asked her what she wanted in terms of positive change. She said that she had heard good reports about our form of craniosacral therapy, and "wanted to relax more."

She went on to say that she had a diagnosis of bipolar disorder and had been in and out of the psychiatric hospital regularly over the last twenty years. She said that she experienced periods of lethargy followed by periods of hectic activity.

In Denmark some hospitals have a somewhat flexible system of psychiatric care. After patients are admitted and have been treated for a while, they can ask the psychiatrist to be discharged when they feel that they can cope, and later can be re-admitted when they feel that is needed. This client told me that when she was not in a depressed state, she felt compelled to action, to the point of being frantic to get everything done. Then, when she collapsed into depression, she would have herself hospitalized.

When this woman told me her history, I could read in her body language that she was dissociated, and this was confirmed by her words. Rather than being grounded and at ease in her body, she said she felt as if she were looking at her life from the outside as it passed in front of her.

Many women experience postpartum (after childbirth) depression, and this woman's bipolar states had started shortly after the birth of her son. It's not unusual for postpartum depression to provoke a crisis in a woman's marriage as well as in herself; because of the wife's dorsal branch-induced shutdown/depression, the husband might feel that she is no longer the same woman he fell in love with. This particular couple's life took an unfortunate turn for the worse, as the birth of their baby did not bring them the joy they had dreamed of.

Postpartum depression can be exacerbated if the birth was difficult, especially if it resulted in a cesarean section. Even when a C-section is necessary for medical reasons to save the life of the child or mother, it is still a shock for the woman's body, and leaves scar tissue not only in the muscles of the abdomen but also in the uterus. It can take years for a woman to get over postpartum depression and, unfortunately, some women never do.

I told this woman that I was not qualified to treat her psychiatric condition, but that I would try to help her relax by making her autonomic nervous system more flexible. As a body therapist, I am careful not to imply that I can successfully treat any psychiatric problem. If a patient has a psychiatric diagnosis and I do not feel totally comfortable treating them, I sometimes decide not to. If you are a therapist and you are ever in doubt in such a case, you can always ask the client to consult with their own psychiatrist or psychologist to determine whether there is any reason that you should not treat them.

I found that this client's first two cervical vertebrae were rotated, and that she might benefit if we could improve the function of the ventral branch of her vagus nerve. I showed her how to do the Basic Exercise to improve the position of these vertebrae. Afterwards, when I checked her again, the first two vertebrae of her neck were less rotated, and her ventral vagus nerve was functional.

A week later, when the woman came back for her next session, she seemed like another person; she was calm and centered. I checked her vagal function and the position of her first two vertebrae. These were still good; the effects of the first treatment had held. She told me that she now had good energy and was getting things done, but that she did them calmly. She said that she felt confident and ready to get on with her life again.

I felt that we had solved the issue in her nervous system. She had been bipolar, moving back and forth between agitated states of stress and collapsed states of dorsal vagal withdrawal, without finding her way into social engagement. Now that she was coming from a state of social engagement, she felt robust, and her nervous system was flexible. She could be stressed or shut down temporarily, and return to social engagement when the challenge passed.

I told her that she was welcome to come back if she thought that she needed help again. I advised her to go to a good psychologist, and suggested that she could use help to manage her relationships in a new way and structure her plans for her future.

By now, her son had grown up; he was attending school and living on his own. My client expressed regret over missing much of the experience of being a mother because she had spent so much time in the psychiatric hospital. Over the twenty years since giving birth, she had also missed opportunities for an education, a career, and a meaningful job. She was also living with a man who had fit into her life as long as she was manic-depressive, but their relationship no longer worked for her.

She was not sad, however, but quietly optimistic. She was neither manic nor depressed when she assessed her situation; she was calm and spoke in a clear voice as she expressed her determination to make a good, meaningful life for herself.

ADHD and Hyperactivity

In addition to chronic stimulation of the sympathetic nervous system in children with attention deficit hyperactivity disorder (ADHD), I believe that there may be another physical cause.

I had five clients—all boys with ADHD—during the same period of time, and noticed that all five had hiatal hernias.[81] This led me to speculate that the reason they continually moved from one position to another was to change the level of tension in their respiratory diaphragm. After a few seconds in the new position, that would also become uncomfortable, so they needed to move again.

I was able to ease their symptoms with a combination of two techniques. The Basic Exercise addressed a dysfunction in the vagus nerve, allowing the upper third of the esophagus to relax. This then allowed the hiatal hernia technique to gently stretch the esophagus so that the stomach could free itself from the respiratory diaphragm and drop to its normal position.

Many people are diagnosed by a psychologist or psychiatrist without any consideration that their problems might arise from a dysfunction of their autonomic nervous system. It is my experience that bringing the person into a ventral vagal state often causes their problems to diminish or disappear.

CHAPTER 7

Autism Spectrum Disorders

The term autism spectrum disorders (ASD) includes autism, Asperger's syndrome, and other conditions. (ADHD is not defined as an autism spectrum disorder.) ASD encompasses a wide range of symptoms, levels of impairment, and disabilities that can appear in children or adults. These symptoms, assumed to be developmental brain disorders, can cause significant social, behavioral, and communication challenges. However, there are no neural tests for these disorders.

There are many different categories of autism. The disorders affect each person in a unique way, and range from very mild to severe. People with autism spectrum disorders share some of the same symptoms, and seem to handle information in their brain differently than other people do. The exact causes of autism spectrum disorders are unknown. Research suggests that both genes and environment play important roles.

The evidence pointing to genes is based in part on the observation that if one identical twin is autistic, there is a good chance that the other twin will be as well. However, despite spending hundreds of millions of dollars, researchers have yet to identify which genes may be defective in cases of autism. Ideally, this will be determined soon, but at present there is no promising cure for autism spectrum disorder based on genetic research.

Autism-spectrum diagnoses are based primarily on psychologists' observations of behavior. However, the people doing the testing do not usually consider the physiological signs of the social-engagement portion of the autonomic nervous system. But the autonomic nervous system in part determines the emotional state, and the emotional state is a contributing factor in determining behavior. I believe that if we change a person's emotional state, we can change their behavior.

Might some cases of autism spectrum disorder be understood as manifestations of autonomic nervous system disorder? These individuals are often in a chronic state of either fight-or-flight or dorsal vagal withdrawal. Sometimes, for no apparent reason, they shift suddenly from one of these states to another, catching caretakers off guard. Their behavior is frequently unpredictable and inappropriate for the situation.

Based on my clinical experience, I suggest that autism-spectrum tests should include evaluation of the function of their ventral vagus nerve. If it shows dysfunction, further research could tell whether bringing the patient into a state of social engagement by optimizing the function of this nerve brings about positive changes in their behavior. It is my belief that this would be the case.

HOW PREVALENT IS AUTISM?

The increasing number of individuals diagnosed with autism spectrum disorders makes this the most rapidly growing developmental disability, with a 10- to 17-percent annual increase in the United States. About one in sixty-eight children have been identified with ASD, according to estimates from the CDC's Autism and Developmental Disabilities Monitoring Network (ADDM).[82] According to other estimates, autism-spectrum disorders affect one out of ninety children.[83]

The economic costs of autism are also enormous, not only for the individual families but also for society as a whole, as demands for autism-related health care and other services skyrocket. The cost of autism over an average lifespan is $2.4 million per individual in the United States,[84] for an annual total of $20 billion.[85] Other estimates of the cost of supporting children with autism in the U.S. are $61–66 billion a year; for autistic adults, these costs have been estimated at $175–196 billion a year.[86]

More importantly, there is also a human loss to our society. Among the personal costs of autism is the heavy emotional toll it exacts on the parents, which cannot be calculated in dollars. Before the child was born, the parents had dreams and hopes of having a family like other families, with well-functioning children; often autistic individuals cannot hold a job and contribute to the workforce, or can have difficulty in parenting the next generation. Whatever their goals may have been before, the family must now prioritize caring for their child in a new way.

AUTISM AND THE AUTONOMIC NERVOUS SYSTEM

Activity of the spinal sympathetic chain, and/or dorsal vagal activity, can be physiological characteristics of the nervous system of people with various diagnoses on the autism spectrum. They might also have a physical issue arising from a dysfunction in their organs.

Their family or caregivers might notice that people with autism sometimes react with fear and panic even with no apparent reason. They may be hypersensitive, reacting to a stimulus in the environment that other people do not notice, or to something that reminds them of something in their past—or they might simply be imagining something dangerous. Other people looking at their behavior objectively find that these reactions are unfounded and feel there is nothing to be upset about.

Sometimes people on the autism spectrum are trapped in states of fight-or-flight or shutdown, or shift between these two states. They may be in a state of shutdown, folded into themselves and apathetic one moment, then suddenly extroverted, afraid, or aggressive in the next. To others who do not understand their behavior, they react in seemingly strange, unpredictable ways that often make them seem asocial in their behavior. Many parents or caregivers are confused and surprised by these sudden shifts in behavior because they are not aware of anything that could be causing the emotional changes.

Psychological testing for autism evaluates behavior and defines different kinds of autism, but does not consider the underlying physiological factors in terms of Porges's new interpretation of the function of the autonomic nervous system. As a result, treatments have mostly focused on training the parents to try to adapt their behavior to fit the special needs of their child, rather than improving the child's condition so that they do not have these special needs.

The Polyvagal Theory presents a new biobehavioral model linking autistic behavior to specific physiological states of the autonomic nervous system. This allows us the possibility to develop more effective strategies for treating autism.

When we see that many of these individuals are being affected by their spinal sympathetic chain or dorsal vagal activity, or are vacillating between the two, we can simply say that they are not socially engaged. Then we can focus on using or developing interventions that help them to be socially engaged and improve the function of the ventral branch of their vagus nerve and the other four associated cranial nerves—resulting in more social behaviors.

Stephen Porges chose to work with autistic children, and has had success in improving the behavior of many of them. He interpreted this as a verification that there was some validity to the model of the nervous system presented in the Polyvagal Theory. I was inspired by his work and have also been treating autistic individuals with some success.

Hope for Autism: The Listening Project Protocol

Important distinctions were made by Stephen Porges in his Polyvagal Theory and Listening Project that point to specialized functions of the cranial nerves that go to muscles in the middle ear, and to how proper listening enables social engagement.[87]

Porges made a breakthrough in our understanding of hearing, one of the problems affecting about 60 percent of autistic children. I heard Stephen Porges describe this in a lecture at the Breath of Life Conference in London (May 23–24, 2009). He described how problems associated with listening and processing human voices might be related to poor function of cranial nerves V and VII—rather than cranial nerve VIII, as in typical deafness—and how the mechanisms involved in listening may be an important part of autistic symptomology.

People on the autism spectrum are a challenge in many ways to parents, teachers, and other caregivers. Anyone working with autistic children notices that they often do not seem to be able to understand what other people are saying, and cannot carry on normal two-way communication. Many people on the autism spectrum do not seem to understand the meaning of what is being said to them, and many of them do not speak at all. This is especially challenging for psychologists and psychiatrists because autistic individuals usually have difficulty communicating verbally, so that verbally based therapies are not helpful.

Therefore, as a standard practice, their cranial nerve VIII (auditory nerve), which has sensory fibers deep in the inner ear, is tested to find out whether their hearing is sufficient. Most individuals on the autism spectrum pass the standard hearing test, which is usually administered in a quiet room with no background noise, or with the subject wearing headphones that eliminate all sounds other than the frequencies being tested.

The problem with this test for individuals on the autism spectrum is that it only measures part of the auditory mechanism. Stephen Porges realized that for people to hear and understand what is being said, they need two other cranial nerves: the trigeminal nerve (cranial nerve V) and the facial nerve (cranial nerve VII).

In order to learn to speak, we first need to be able to hear and understand spoken language. Porges found that many individuals on the autism spectrum have a dysfunction in cranial nerves V and VII, which interferes with their ability to hear and understand spoken language. These nerves originate in the brainstem, and each has several branches with different functions, two of which go to two muscles in the middle ear. CN VII goes to the stapedius, a tiny muscle in the middle ear, and CN V goes to the *tensor tympani,* at the eardrum.

One of the many functions of cranial nerve CN VII is innervation of the stapedius muscle. When the stapedius functions properly, it helps to reduce the volume of sounds that are above and below the frequency range of the human female voice, to help a child focus on sounds in the frequency range of a mother's voice. When this muscle functions properly, a child can easily hear its mother's voice above background noise, learn language from its mother, and communicate with her and other people.

CN VII, which innervates the stapedius muscle, has other branches as well, one of which controls the muscles of the face (which have been referred to as "organs of emotional expression"). When this nerve is not functioning properly, there is often a lack of facial expression. One characteristic of both children and adults with a diagnosis of autism is a lack of natural facial expression; their flat facial affect makes it difficult for people to read their emotions in a conversation. Because of this, other people tend to think that the autistic individual lacks empathy.

There is a neurological connection between proper hearing and the muscles that open the eyes. The flat ring muscle around the eye is innervated by the seventh cranial nerve, and people with hearing problems often have drooping eyelids. Lifting the eyebrows— the way we do when something just heard is an "eye-opener"—can help us understand spoken language. All these factors point to the importance to hearing of the proper functioning of the seventh cranial nerve.

A branch of CN V regulates the tension in the *tensor tympani* muscle, which is involved in regulating the Eustachian tube that connects to the throat. The *tensor tympani* is similar to the stapedius, regulating the rigidity of the ossicles (small middle-ear bones). Tensing the ossicle chain increases the tension of the eardrum, diminishing the volume of low-frequency background sounds.

One of the roles of the stapedius and *tensor tympani* muscles is to dampen sounds such as those produced by chewing. If the middle-ear muscles do not contract sufficiently, the perceived volume of low-frequency sounds can be extremely high, and even mask human-voice sounds. This condition is called *hyperacusis*. For people suffering from this condition, incoming sounds can be disturbing or even painful. Some autistic children put their fingers in their ears to block out sounds, especially low-frequency sounds.

In this condition, a child processes acoustic information only within a restricted frequency range, so that sounds in the frequency band of human speech may be lost in background sounds, while lower-pitched sounds may be functionally amplified. Children with hypersensitivity to sound might overreact to other people's voices, especially the low-pitched voices of some men. And when they put their fingers in their ears, this may be misinterpreted to mean that the child does not want to listen to what is being said, when in actuality they are just trying to protect their ears from a painful experience.

Everyday noises that include low frequencies (e.g., vacuum cleaners, traffic, or escalators) seem unbearably loud to people with this condition. They cannot understand what is being said to them due to background noises that bother them tremendously, even though the same noises do not bother other people.

One of my patients, an eleven-year-old boy, stuffed his fingers into his ears to reduce the sound whenever a train went by at some distance from my office window. I had never noticed the sound of the trains passing before, and my other clients never seemed to react to it.

A different kind of dysfunction of the muscles and nerves can result in an opposite kind of problem with hearing and understanding what is being said. Muscle tone may be insufficient to amplify the sound adequately, so that not enough sound gets through, and the child can appear to be deaf to what is being said to him. This is often misinterpreted as a lack of interest in communication and social activity, or taken to mean that the child does not want to respond or do what is being requested of him.

Sometimes children with these problems can become very skilled at reading lips and interpreting body language. They may appear to be able to carry on a conversation and to be sociable—but they have a problem if the person who is speaking is not directly in front of them so that they cannot read their lips.

Some adults also struggle to understand what is being said unless they can see the other person's face. People who are lip-reading fixate their gaze on the other person's mouth, unlike a person with normal hearing who looks into the other person's eyes, or looks away while listening. Adults who have difficulty understanding if more than one person talks simultaneously may avoid going to parties or crowded restaurants, preferring to meet people one on one. Or they may use another strategy—talking all the time, to avoid revealing that they cannot understand others.

Children on the autism spectrum can have major difficulties functioning normally in a noisy classroom. When a child is overly sensitive to sound, a high level of background noise can be painful, while children with a normally functioning inner ear find the same level of noise acceptable.

For a child with severe hyperacusis, environmental sounds cause bursts of pain that they cannot escape. Going through the various soundscapes of daily life might feel like the experience of rats in a cage being stressed by electrical shocks at unpredictable time intervals. The children might not even realize that they have a problem; if they were born with hyperacusis, they might not know that their randomly traumatic experience is not normal, and might just assume, "That's life."

Imagine watching a movie with the soundtrack turned up full blast—the actors' voices are screaming at you, and you cannot wait to get out of the theater. You leave, holding your ears. But what if you were an autistic child who cannot get out of the cinema?

In order to investigate the implications of cranial nerve dysfunction—and ultimately to prove the validity of the Polyvagal Theory—Stephen Porges designed his Listening Project Protocol for a research program that he carried out with subjects on the autism spectrum.[88] In peer-reviewed research, he describes his empirical studies using the Listening Project Protocol with autistic children (see below).

Porges's research and scientific articles over the last twenty years have broken new ground in treating autistic conditions. Identifying a physiological pattern that may be partly responsible for autistic behavioral patterns is a significant breakthrough in our understanding of autism, and has opened possibilities for new forms of treatment. The method that he developed has already helped many people to improve their communication skills and social behavior.

Porges hypothesized that the reason many children on the autism spectrum have difficulty in using language to interact is dysfunction in the neural regulation of their middle-ear muscles, described above. CN V and CN VII, two of the cranial nerves necessary for social engagement, originate in the brainstem and have branches that go to those two muscles in the middle ear.

Porges treated a large group of children with a diagnosis of autism using an ingenious therapeutic intervention. In Porges's Listening Project Protocol research, all of the children tested had diagnoses on the autism spectrum, and many of them also had hyperacusis. All of the children, after receiving extensive hearing tests, received five forty-five-minute sessions daily for five days.

In one publication, Porges and his group demonstrated that specially computer-altered music improved auditory processing skills and increased ventral vagal regulation of the heart.[89]

A second publication describes two trials conducted by Porges's team. One trial contrasted a group of children wearing headphones only with another group receiving computer-altered music, processed with an algorithm to enhance the acoustic features of prosody. In the second trial, one group received the computer-altered music and the other group received the same music, but unaltered. In both trials, only the group receiving the computer-altered music exhibited a reduction in auditory hypersensitivity.[90]

I had a chance to hear the special music myself. After I listened for a few minutes, I felt as if my middle-ear muscles had been stimulated and exercised. My eardrum itched, and the structures in my middle ear felt as if they were hopping, dancing, and vibrating. More importantly, I experienced an improvement in my hearing and in my ability to hear speech more clearly.

At his lectures, Porges presented inspiring videos showing some of the changes in the children and how, when they could understand what was being said, they emerged from their previous social isolation and began to relate to others. Porges is constantly working on improving the acoustic stimulation that he uses, and the means of delivering it. At the time of this writing, in 2016, he was conducting registered clinical trials in Melbourne, Los Angeles, and Toronto.

The Role of Hearing in Autism Spectrum Disorders

In order to be sociable and carry on a two-way communication, people have to hear and interpret the meaning of words spoken by others. As described above, problems with hearing and understanding characterize many individuals on the autism spectrum. This phenomenon is well recognized; Stephen Porges initially pointed this out in his presentation of the Polyvagal Theory, and I have confirmed it in my practice. However, these hearing problems are most often related to a dysfunctional CN V and CN VII (as Porges discovered) and not CN VIII, the auditory nerve, often incorrectly assumed to be exclusively responsible for hearing.

When an autistic, Asperger's, or otherwise challenging child comes to my clinic, I ask the parents about their child's hearing. Invariably, they say that their child's hearing was tested by an ear specialist who reported that it was normal. Most autistic children have their hearing tested in the usual way: they wear headphones, and respond when they hear the varied volumes and frequencies of sound from the headphones.

The parents are almost always told that their child has good hearing, but this misses the core of the autistic child's hearing problem. It is not a question of the child hearing single tones in a test, without background noises. The question should be: can the child hear the human voice in the presence of background noise? Does the child have the ability to filter out background sounds, especially low-frequency sounds?

One mother brought her nine-year-old son to me because of his aggressive behavior at school. I usually do my own simple test to check such a patient's ability to hear well. I ask the child to turn around, so that their back is turned and they cannot read my lips. Then I give them a simple task to perform—for example, to put their coat on.

Often the parent will protest, saying that this puts the child at a dis-advantage since it's easiest for them when they can see the speaker's face. This particular mother said something similar. So I asked her what happens when her son is in the next room or does not see her face, and she tries to get him to do something that she wants.

"If he does not answer," the mother responded, "I stay calm and tell him again."

"If he still does not answer, what do you do?"

She replied, "I tell him a third time. If he still does not do it, I know it is because he doesn't want to answer me. Sometimes I get so irritated that I slap him."

From her son's point of view, he was occupied doing something and was not aware of the mother's message because his fifth and seventh cranial nerves were not functioning sufficiently to filter out background sounds. He was probably not even aware that his mother was talking to him. Then, all of a sudden, without his understanding why, his mother would slap him, and yell at him in an angry voice.

Even though she had told him something three times, he had been unable to hear and understand what she said. In her own frustration at not being heard, she then slapped him, but from his perspective this was without warning; he did not know what led up to the slap. So he might logically interpret his mother's message as, "If you want another person's attention, hit them, and then give them your message."

Sometimes, when the boy was in school and asked one of the other children to do something, and if the other child did not do it right away, he would slap them without warning to get their attention. It is no wonder that this child had a hard time playing with other children. His mother had inadvertently taught him this antisocial pattern herself.

In my clinic, when children turn their back to me and do not respond to my simple request to put their coats on, I do not assume that they heard and understood it just because I said it. Instead, I suspect dysfunction of CN V and VII. If this is indeed the case, and autistic individuals cannot understand what others are saying, they will of course have a hard time recognizing how to use language to get others to understand and help them.

THE EVOLUTION OF HEARING

Early in the evolution of Earth's creatures, large predators including the dinosaurs and other great lizards roamed the land, often preying upon small mammals. The largest animals that could threaten these dinosaurs and lizards pounded the earth with their feet when they walked or ran, producing low-frequency percussive sounds. The dinosaurs registered these low-frequency vibrations in the nerve endings wrapping their large skeletal bones.

Information about the approach of a potential predator was crucial, especially for protection of their offspring. But these large creatures could not hear sounds in higher frequencies. Paleontologists have found that their middle-ear bones were attached to the jawbone, unlike those of later species. Thus it is speculated that dinosaurs "heard" by registering low-frequency vibrations in the bones of their skeleton, but could not hear higher-frequency sounds made by mammals.

Mammals have evolved ears that allow us to hear higher frequencies; our middle-ear bones, detached from our jaws, vibrate based on sonic waves in the air. Mammalian "voices" are in a higher frequency range than the rumblings of the dinosaurs and large lizards. Therefore early mammals were able to communicate with each other without being detected by the larger and faster animals that were their predators, and this was a potential advantage in their struggle for survival.

However, if mammals indiscriminately let all the sounds of their environment into their ears, including both very high and low frequencies, we would experience a confusing cacophony. The higher and lower frequencies would drown out the mammalian-voice sounds. For humans, sounds in the vital frequency range of the female voice might convey information from the mother that is crucial to a child's survival in a dangerous situation.

So how does our hearing focus on these important frequencies? The ability of mammals to filter out sounds depends on varying levels of tension in the stapedius and *tensor tympani* muscles in the middle ear. These effectively block out both high- and low-frequency sounds, leaving only the sounds roughly in the range of the human voice. A well-functioning stapedius muscle can filter out sounds above and below the range of the human voice—even otherwise deafeningly loud noises.[91]

The evolution of the structures of the ear and the sense of hearing is well documented in the field of evolutionary biology, from the time of the early dinosaurs starting 190 million years ago until today. In mammals, three small parts of the jawbone became separated from the rest of the jaw. These three small bones as a group are called the ossicles. (The root *os-* means "bone," and *ossicle* means "tiny bone.") These three bones are called the hammer *(malleus)*, the anvil *(incus)*, and the stirrup *(stapes)* because they resemble these shapes. They are enjoined in synovial joints, and held together by a ligament in a flexible "chain."

Movement of the ossicles is controlled (either facilitated or restricted) by adjustments in the tension of the *tensor tympani* and stapedius muscles, which attach to the ossicles at opposite ends of the chain. These muscles affect the hearing in different ways. The tympanic membrane (eardrum) is round in shape, like a drumhead; the *tensor tympani* muscle connects it to the malleus, one of the ossicles.

Changes in tension in the *tensor tympani* muscle determine how much the eardrum can vibrate. Sounds are louder with increased tension. The *tensor tympani* is innervated by a branch of the fifth cranial nerve, and acts as a kind of volume control on how much sound gets passed on to the receptors of the acoustic nerve deep in the auditory canal.

The stapedius, about one millimeter long, is the tiniest muscle in the entire body. It is innervated by a motor branch of the seventh cranial nerve, which changes the level of muscle tension. The stapedius is also a very thin muscle. It originates in a small cavity surrounding the bones of the middle ear, and inserts into the neck of the stapes (one of the three ossicles). The stapedius only transmits certain frequency ranges as it tenses and relaxes. With normal hearing, the sound frequencies of the human female voice get through easily, while sounds above and below these frequencies are largely filtered out.

To register the changes of frequency when someone else is talking requires a well-functioning stapedius muscle in order to separate out the range of sounds needed for us to hear, understand, and communicate with each other. This function is crucial for a child in learning vocabulary and the melody of language.

TREATING HEARING IN AUTISTIC CHILDREN

A characteristic common to people who are socially engaged is that we usually have a melodic voice that can communicate feeling. This voice melody, or prosody, makes it easier for other people to understand us. In contrast, people with autism often have a flat, monotonous voice, which can verge on sounding mechanical and robotic.

Perhaps the reason that they lack prosody in their voice is that they cannot hear it in other people's voices due to a dysfunctional CN VII. If a child cannot hear and appreciate, or feel the emotions communicated by, the melody in the voices of others, they cannot comprehend the benefits of using melody in their own voice, much less learn to express it.

This quality of the voice is not primarily a vocal problem per se. As soon as we help people on the autism spectrum to a state of social engagement through improved function of their cranial nerves, the quality of their voice changes; they immediately have more prosody, and it is easier for others to understand what they are saying.

Sometimes hearing can be improved with the Basic Exercise by increasing the flow of blood to the brainstem, where cranial nerves V and VII originate. The Basic Exercise can also release tension between the base of the cranium (where the nucleus of CN V is located) and the first three vertebrae. The Neuro-Fascial Release Technique can also be sufficient to reset the function of these nerves and improve social behavior.

With the understanding gained from my study of the Polyvagal Theory, I developed my own approach to autism spectrum disorders. I evaluate the function of cranial nerves V, VII, IX, X, and XI, and then I use a selection of specific biomechanical cranial techniques to release restrictions and enable proper function in these nerves.

Based on my clinical experiences and the feedback of my students, I have confirmed that it is possible to improve the communication skills of some people with a diagnosis of autism. Several of my patients who originally came to me with an autism diagnosis were evaluated again after I treated them and were found to be no longer autistic.

I have learned over the years to be careful about saying "cure autism," usually simply stating that I have helped some people with a diagnosis of autism to improve their hearing and achieve more empathy and better communication skills. Many professionals working in the field believe that autism cannot be cured and are more receptive to a claim that it is possible in many cases to improve communication.

Treating Autism

Over the years, I have successfully helped many children and young people with a diagnosis on the autism spectrum. Many such children have problems with normal social behavior; they do not seem interested in other people, avoiding looking at them or making eye contact. They seem to lack empathy, and would rather spend time alone or playing on their electronic devices.

Their parents may designate other young people as "friends" if they can sit together in the same room for periods of time. However, the children do not really interact with these friends, but sit in their own worlds, playing alongside each other but by themselves.

Some autistic individuals lack verbal communication skills, and cannot take part in a meaningful two-way conversation. They do not seem able to listen or understand what is being said, and they are not playful. Some do not speak at all; others, when they do speak, may repeat like a parrot what was just said by someone else, or repeat sentences from a movie. Sometimes they continue speaking without pausing for the other person to respond.

To start to make sense of all the various behaviors exhibited by individuals on the autism spectrum, I have observed that such individuals are not socially engaged, and have faulty neuroception. I have been able to help some of them by getting them into a state of social engagement. In several instances, I have brought about normal vagal function and improved the function of the other four cranial nerves involved in social engagement. This brought the individuals out of states of stress or dorsal vagal withdrawal and spontaneously improved their communication skills.

Perhaps one of my most unexpected discoveries in doing body therapy is that I have found tension in the right sternocleidomastoid (SCM) muscle—and an accompanying deformation of the skull called "flat back of the head" or plagiocephaly—in every client diagnosed with ADHD or a diagnosis on the autism spectrum. Research published in the journal *Pediatrics* reported that this deformation of the skull, usually only on one side, is present in a higher percentage of children with autism and ADHD, compared to normally functioning children.[92]

The sternocleidomastoid muscle is attached to the base of the temporal bone, on the side of the skull, so that chronic tension in the SCM muscle noticeably deforms the shape of the skull in a particular way. Although this client group consists mostly of children and young people, this deformation of the skull is not confined to children; I also see it in many adults who have had difficulties being socially engaged. This same approach can achieve similar improvements in adults.

Can certain characteristic shapes of the skull put pressure on certain blood vessels or nerves inside the skull? A baby's cranium is made up of several plates, connected by tough connective tissue. A constant pull on the temporal bone from chronic tension in the SCM muscle can pull the baby's cranium out of shape. If the tension in the muscle is not released, the skull remains out of shape as the child matures.

Many parents come to me because they already know that their child has a flat back of the head. If the parents were not already aware of it, I show them how to feel the shape of their child's head, and to notice any asymmetry there before we start the treatment. Relaxing the tension in the sternocleidomastoid muscle on one side often gives a noticeable improvement in the shape of the child's head within a few minutes.

Technique for Rounding a Flat Back of the Head

I start by feeling the two sternocleidomastoid muscles, and I work on the side that is tighter. I take the top of the child's SCM muscle on that side firmly but gently between my thumb and index finger. This must not cause pain. (See "Sternocleidomastoid" in the Appendix.) I ask one of the parents to hold the foot on the side where we are going to release the SCM, and to gently bend their child's foot down at the ankle joint with one hand, and then with their second hand to bend their child's toes up. After a minute or two, the child relaxes and the sternocleidomastoid muscle is much more relaxed and pliable. When the SCM no longer pulls on one side of the back of the cranium, the part that was flat fills out, becomes rounded, and the two sides become symmetrical. The rationale behind this technique is found in Tom Myers' book *Anatomy Trains,* in which he describes the "superficial front line."[93]

Then the parent and I evaluate the back of the child's head again. It has always become more symmetrical. When the child comes back for another treatment, I observe that the changes have held.

AUTISM: A CASE STUDY

As exciting as it was for me to see the changes in the children that I treated, and to hear about their improvements, the next step was to find out whether other people could learn the approach and have similar success. In my school in Copenhagen, we offered a two-year program based on the biomechanical cranial techniques I had learned from my teacher, Alain Gehin. For many years, I started the first day of the first course teaching students my Neuro-Fascial Release Technique (see Part Two). In this way I began to realize how simple and powerful this technique is.

On the second day, I asked whether any of the students had tried the techniques they learned and, if so, what they experienced. One young man named Thor told the class of his success. He had gone home with the idea of reviewing the techniques that he had learned that first day, and treated his younger brother, William, who had had a diagnosis of infantile autism and was then seventeen years old.

William was asocial, and sat in his chair looking down at his PlayStation or playing with his keys. He did not speak or make eye contact with anyone. He could also be moody; if he was upset about something, even though it might seem trivial to other people, he would withdraw into himself and sulk. Thor told of one mute episode that lasted for three months after William was made to wear a T-shirt that he did not want to wear. Even though he only wore T-shirt for one day, he sulked in silence for three months.

After Thor did the Neuro-Fascial Release Technique on him, William sat back and looked Thor in the eyes, which he had not done before. Then he stood up and balanced on one foot. Like many people with autism,

William had been unable to balance well enough to stand on one foot. Then he shifted his weight to the other foot, and stood on that. That one technique was enough for William to be brought into a state of social engagement. He started to communicate with his family and other students at school, and started making friends.

Thor asked me to also treat William, and I treated him four or five times. But most of the work on his nervous system had been done by Thor's treatments before William ever came to me.

Over the next few months, William made many friends, traveled to other European countries on vacations, got involved in theater, took yoga classes, and started dating. He went on to finish a bachelor's degree from Copenhagen University in the Study of Media, and then to receive a master's degree.

The last time I saw William, he told me that he is doing very well, and proudly related that he had taken a vacation to Amsterdam with three of his friends, also young adults with challenging diagnoses. They had handled the whole trip themselves—booked a hotel, found restaurants, visited museums, and had a good time together and enjoyed the trip. William had attained ranking as a chess master, and he had beaten several other international chess masters. He is also just starting an apprenticeship as a sound designer for a Danish software company that produces video games.

You can see Thor tell William's story on YouTube (Search "autism, William, Stanley").

SPECIAL CONSIDERATIONS IN TREATING AUTISTIC CHILDREN

Treating children (especially those on the autism spectrum) with hands-on techniques has its special challenges. Even children without autism will usually not lie still on a massage table for very long. Those with medical histories have often had a history of countless visits to doctors and hospitals, where they have been forced to lie still for an examination, or to receive painful injections.

It is hard to imagine how a child with negative experiences like that can feel safe, especially on the first treatment—lying on her back in a position of total helplessness, in an unfamiliar room, and being approached by a complete stranger who towers over her and starts doing something to her. Resistance is understandably triggered by this, and it takes patience, skill, and experience on the part of the therapist to help these children feel safe.

Many autistic children, furthermore, do not like being touched. A treatment is often an improvised dance of the child, the parent, and me before I can gain the child's confidence enough for him to relax on the table and allow me to get my hands on him so that I can treat him. I find that succeeding with an autistic child, however, is always deeply rewarding.

If you are treating autistic children, there are a few things that you should know. When they come into your space for the first time, it is natural for them to feel unsafe. They do not know you, and they often react with fear upon seeing the massage table, which looks like a medical examination table. You may have the best of therapeutic intentions, but they do not know that. If you or their parents hold them down, it is counterproductive; they will feel even more threatened, and perhaps violated.

All children can be wary of being touched, especially by a stranger. A lot of these patients have pain in their head and neck, where I want to work. Perhaps they will allow me to touch their knee or elbow, but push my hands away when I try to touch their head or neck. The techniques that I choose must therefore be highly effective, since there is such a small window of opportunity in which I can touch these children, especially at the start of their very first session.

I must first make them feel safe, and this might not happen at all on the initial treatment. I might give the child toys to play with, and wait until they have their attention on the toy, or I'll have their parent lie on the table next to them, maybe even with the child on their stomach. I keep eye contact with the child, and when I see any expression of pain or discomfort, I pause in what I am doing and let the child relax before I go further.

My cardinal rule in treating children, especially autistic children, is that they must feel safe, and must be respected, every step of the way. This is a prerequisite to certain techniques in particular that help the child's nervous system.

In my clinic, when I schedule a child for their first treatment, I like to talk with one of the parents on the phone first; I do not like to talk about the child's "problems" in front of the child. I tell parents not to have high expectations for the first session, and that I might not even be able to touch their child, much less do a technique, the first time. I inform them that my practice is to respect the child's resistance on the first session, and not push beyond their comfort zone. Also, I tell the parents that they should not try to help me by forcing their child to lie still.

If the child has a good first or second session with me (including attaining a more symmetrical and rounded back of the cranium—see "Technique for Rounding a Flat Back of the Head" on page 178) he will more readily accept another session and be more willing to lie still and allow me to work on him. Rather than reacting to me with fear and panic, he will often look at me and smile. I feel that this is significant, since one of the characteristics of children on the autism spectrum is that they usually avoid looking at others, making eye contact, or smiling.

One problem for autistic individuals who lack normal two-way verbal communication is that they cannot understand the spoken word well enough to know what to expect in a therapeutic encounter. While the value of the therapy may be obvious to their parents or to health care professionals, autistic children may have no understanding of why they are there, or the value they might gain from the treatment. They most likely have no idea that there is even anything wrong with them, or that their life can be better.

Their behavior changes, however, when they realize that they are safe with you, especially once your treatment makes them feel better.

Concluding Remarks

While the Polyvagal Theory has given me increased clarity and understanding in regard to treating various difficult emotional, physical, and mental conditions, the insights I've gained into treatment of individuals on the autism spectrum have quite possibly been the most profound.

A common characteristic of people on the autistic spectrum is that they have difficulty communicating normally, not only with people in their everyday life, but also with their caregivers and with people trying to treat them. These communication difficulties limit the possibilities in their lives, as well as the efforts of others to communicate with them and to treat them. This causes suffering for them and their families. Understandably, their caregivers often feel helpless, challenged, and not up to the task. Helping individuals on the autistic spectrum is a journey into a vast, uncharted area.

For caregivers and therapists, trying to grasp the idiosyncrasies of behavior exhibited by those on the autism spectrum may only add to the confusion. However, when we observe autistic individuals from the point of view of the Polyvagal Theory, we realize that we may be able to help by simply improving the person's ventral vagal function.

At any given moment, a person can be in only one of the three autonomic states. Autism-spectrum individuals can suddenly shift between states of stress and withdrawal without others understanding why. Enabling the state of social engagement by improving the function of cranial nerves may have the potential to stabilize these shifts, and reduce some of the difficulty that these individuals commonly experience.

Furthermore, correcting auditory issues by improving the function of the fifth and seventh cranial nerves often leads to dramatic improvement in a person's communication skills, social behaviors, and empathy. Positive changes of this nature tend to build on themselves, further aiding the person's development.

When two people are socially engaged and communicating face to face, they pass information about their emotional states by small movements of facial muscles. This also stimulates the nerves in the muscles of each person's own face, so that their fifth and seventh cranial nerves give them ongoing feedback and a clear idea of what they are feeling themselves and what they feel about the other person.

Our society increasingly relies on emails and text messages. TV anchors often have deadpan faces, or assume put-on expressions. More and more people deaden their faces with Botox, or reduce their expressiveness with plastic surgery. However, the more we communicate without seeing each others' faces and hearing the changes of tone in each other's voices, the more impersonal the interchange will be, and the less we are able to communicate anything emotionally. We can talk, but with words alone we are just passing data.

Telephones are a step up in communication from emails because they capture changes in vocal expression. Skype and FaceTime give us both the sound of the voice and the facial expressions—but nothing beats face-to-face communication.

The less children relate to adults who communicate fully using a melodic voice and an expressive face, the more the children's facial expressivity will be underused and underdeveloped. Is it any wonder that we have increasing numbers of children with autism, ADHD, and other communication disorders?

Beyond relating to autistic people, similar difficulties arise from time to time relating to anyone else in any one of our "normal" relationships. Our interactions with other people would be so very easy if both we and they could be socially engaged all of the time. First, it is helpful to realize that we are not in a ventral vagal state all the time—and neither are they. Second, we now know that we can do something to bring ourselves or the other person into a state of social engagement.

It is my feeling that we have just begun to explore the potential of the Polyvagal Theory not only to help people on the autism spectrum but to help each of us in all of our relationships with others.

EXERCISES TO RESTORE SOCIAL ENGAGEMENT

Part Two explores the healing power of the vagus nerve. Optimal health is possible only when we have a well-functioning ventral branch of the vagus nerve. The exercises and techniques in this part should help most people to move from a state of either chronic spinal sympathetic chain activity (stress) or dorsal vagal activity (shutdown) to a state of social engagement. These exercises can also be used to prevent problems in the autonomic nervous system from developing, and to maintain a general level of well-being.

When you begin to do these exercises for the first time, I suggest that you start a simple journal. Write down any symptoms or issues that bother you. Also, take a look at the many symptoms listed in the "Heads of the Hydra" list at the beginning of Part One. You might want to add one or more of these to your list.

Note how often a given symptom has appeared. For example, your symptom may present "all the time," "every morning," "once a week," or "once a month." If you have a migraine headache every day, your goal is certainly to be totally free of migraines; however, any improvement would be welcomed as a positive result.

Also note how strong your symptoms are. You might write that "They bother me, but I get through the day anyway," "They require me to take medication," "They are so strong that I cannot go to work or take part in normal social activities," "I cannot sleep," or "I cannot get out of bed in the morning." You might prefer to evaluate the pain or symptom using a scale from one to ten.

After you have been doing the exercises, you can look back at your list and note any changes—for example, "The migraines are less frequent," "The pain is less severe," or "I spend less money on painkillers every month." Focus on how the exercises have helped—that you do not have the symptom(s) so often, or that the problem is not so severe. Perhaps whatever symptoms remain will diminish or disappear as you keep doing the exercises.

You might also notice other positive changes—for example, are you sleeping better? Breathing better? Is your appetite more normal? All of these contribute to better health and resiliency.

The Basic Exercise

The goal of this exercise is to enhance social engagement. It repositions the atlas (C1, the first cervical/neck vertebra) and the axis (C2) and increases mobility in the neck and the entire spine. (See "Axis" and "Atlas" in the Appendix.) It increases blood flow to the brainstem, where the five cranial nerves necessary for social engagement originate. This can have a positive effect on the ventral branch of the vagus nerve (CN X), as well as on cranial nerves V, VII, IX, and XI.

The Basic Exercise is effective, easy to learn, and easy to do, and takes less than two minutes to complete. I usually teach this exercise to my clients in their very first session.

BEFORE AND AFTER DOING THE BASIC EXERCISE

Evaluate the relative freedom of movement of your head and neck. Rotate your head to the right as far as it goes comfortably. Then come back to the center, pause, and rotate your head to the left. How far do you rotate to each side? Is there any pain or stiffness?

After doing the exercise, make these same movements again. Is there any improvement in the range of your movement? If there was pain when you rotated your head, did the exercise reduce the level of the pain?

Most people I have treated are surprised to experience an improvement in the range of movement as they rotate their head to the right and left. Better movement of the neck often accompanies an improvement in the circulation of blood to the brainstem, which in turn improves the function of the ventral branch of the vagus nerve.

You or your client will probably want to repeat the exercise as needed.

BASIC EXERCISE INSTRUCTIONS

The first few times that you do the exercise, you should lie on your back. After you are familiar with the exercise, you can do it sitting on a chair, standing, or lying on your back.

1. Lying comfortably on your back, weave the fingers of one hand together with the fingers of the other hand (Figure 4, 5, and 6).

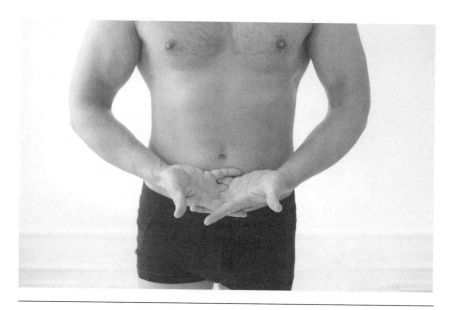

Figure 4. Fingers interwoven

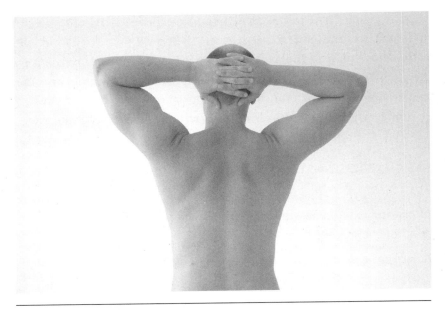

Figure 5. Hands behind the head

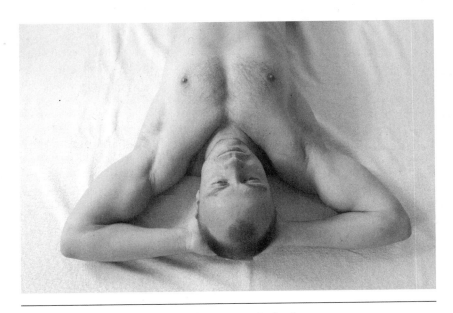

Figure 6. Lying on the back

2. Put your hands behind the back of your head, with the weight of your head resting comfortably on your interwoven fingers. You should feel the hardness of your cranium with your fingers, and you should feel the bones of your fingers on the back of your head. If you have a stiff shoulder and cannot bring both of your hands up behind the back of your head, it is sufficient to use one hand, with the fingers and palm contacting both sides of the back of your head.

3. Keeping your head in place, look to the right, moving only your eyes, as far as you comfortably can. Do not turn your head; just move your eyes. Keep looking to the right (Figure 7).

4. After a short period of time—up to thirty or even sixty seconds— you will swallow, yawn, or sigh. This is a sign of relaxation in your autonomic nervous system. (A normal inbreath is followed by an outbreath, but a sigh is different—after you breathe in, a second inbreath follows on top of the first inbreath, before the outbreath.)

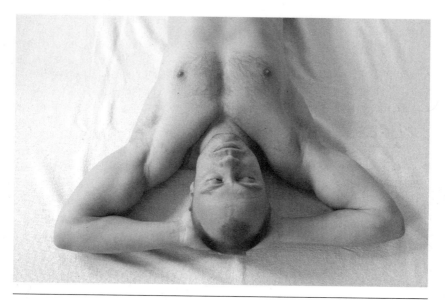

Figure 7. Looking to the right

5. Bring your eyes back to looking straight ahead.

6. Leave your hands in place, and keep your head still. This time, move your eyes to the left (Figure 8).

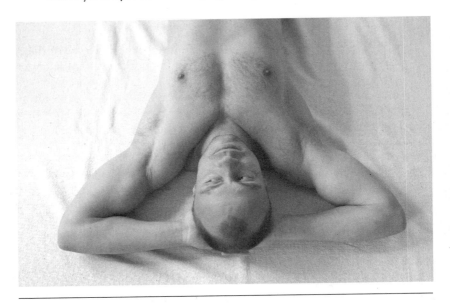

Figure 8. Looking to the left

7. Hold your eyes there until you notice a sigh, a yawn, or a swallow.

Now that you have you have completed the Basic Exercise, take your hands away, and sit up or stand up.

Evaluate what you have experienced. Has there been any improvement in the mobility of your neck? Has your breathing changed? Do you notice anything else?

NOTE: If you become dizzy when you sit up or stand up, it is probably because you relaxed when you were lying down, and your blood pressure dropped. This is a normal reaction. It usually takes a minute or two before your blood pressure adjusts and pumps more blood to your brain.

CERVICAL VERTEBRAE AND VENTRAL VAGAL DYSFUNCTION

When I test clients and find that they have ventral vagal dysfunction, I also observe that they have an upper cervical misalignment—i.e., a rotation of the vertebrae C1 (the atlas) and a tipping of C2 (the axis) away from their optimal positions. Using the Basic Exercise almost always brings my clients back into a better alignment of C1 and C2, and when I test them again I find that they have proper ventral vagal function.

A rotation of C1 and C2 can put pressure on the vertebral artery, which supplies the frontal lobes and the brainstem, where the five nerves necessary for social engagement originate. From my clinical observations, I believe that it only takes one negative thought to bring C1 and C2 out of joint, affecting our posture and physiology.

I demonstrated this a few times in my advanced craniosacral classes. First, I had the students observe the position of my C1. I lay on my back, and my students could determine the position of my C1 by gently placing the pads of their thumbs on its transverse processes. If there was no rotation of C1, their thumbs would be close to horizontal. However, if one thumb was higher than the other, that would indicate a rotation of the vertebra.

At the start of the experiment, a student observed that his thumbs were horizontal. Then I simply thought about something that was disturbing to me. Immediately, the transverse processes of C1 moved; one side went up and the other went down. The position of C1 felt like it had rotated approximately forty-five degrees away from the horizontal, with one side up (anterior) and the other side down (posterior). (Though this observation is counter to the actual anatomical possibilities for C1 alone to rotate, it is what it feels like under your thumbs if you have them lightly monitoring the transverse processes of C1. The only explanation I have is that the rotation must be a complex combination of the repositioning of C1, C2, and C3 taken together. C1 must somehow slide out of the joint so that it can turn even further.)

I found the experience highly unpleasant, since I had to undergo a change of state away from social engagement. The other students in the class could see a change in my breathing, and a loss of color in my face. Then I had my student perform our hands-on technique for myofascial release (see "Neuro-Fascial Release Technique," on page 195) to realign my C1 and C2. These vertebrae did not come back into place as quickly as they had come out of position. He had to repeat the technique several times until C1 was again horizontal. Finally, I felt more like myself.

The rotation of C1 and C2 has evolutionary survival value; it puts pressure on the vertebral artery, reducing blood flow to the brainstem, which affects the function of the five nerves necessary for social engagement. This puts us into a non-ventral vagal state, which in cases of danger can help our survival by shutting off the higher functions when we have to fight or to flee, or when we cannot face the present situation physically or emotionally.

If our neuroception suddenly registers signals from the environment indicating that we are threatened or in danger, this change in our physiology should be instantaneous—and it is. Interestingly enough, although our nervous system is quick to be upset, it takes a longer time to settle down when we are safe again.

It does not require a trauma to affect C1 and C2; the memory of a past event can do the same thing. Brain-scan studies in women with post-traumatic stress disorder show a reduction in blood flow to their brains' frontal lobes when they hear a re-telling of the traumatic events.[94]

Why would a trauma, the memory of a trauma, or even just a negative thought lead to a structural change such as a rotation of C1 and C2? Ten small muscles connect the occipital bone at the base of the skull with C1 and C2. Eight of these muscles are called the suboccipital muscles, and lie on the posterior (back) surface of the vertebrae. Two other muscles, the *rectus capitis lateralis* and the *rectus capitis anterior,* lie on the anterior (front) surface of these same two vertebrae. They are innervated by the occipital nerve, located on the scalp at the back of the head. (See "Suboccipital muscles," "Vertebral arteries," "Suboccipital muscles with vertebra," and "Suboccipital nerve" in the Appendix.) Inappropriate tensions in any of these ten muscles are enough to shift and hold C1 and C2 out of joint.

The transverse processes of each cervical vertebra have openings (called *foramens*, or *foramina*) to accommodate passage of the vertebral arteries. Rotation or tipping of the vertebrae can twist or put pressure on these arteries, reducing the flow of blood, as in a plastic garden hose; if you put a bend in it, you reduce or shut off the flow of water. The amount of blood passing through these vertebral arteries depends on the position of the upper cervical vertebrae in the neck.

When we do the Basic Exercise, we lie with the weight of our head on our fingers. This pressure is enough to stimulate the occipital nerve, causing these muscles to relax and to come into balance with each other. When we do the Basic Exercise, the first two cervical vertebrae move into a better position relative to each other.

When C1 and C2 come back into place, it relieves tension on the vertebral arteries, providing better blood flow to the brain and brainstem, and allows us to return to social engagement. Adequate blood supply to the cranial nerves, brainstem, and brain is necessary for proper function of the social nervous system as well as other bodily functions.

Concurrently, therefore, with realignment of C1 and C2, there is relief of many of the symptoms that we earlier described as the "Heads of the Hydra."

WHY DO WE MOVE OUR EYES IN THE BASIC EXERCISE?

The Basic Exercise involves movement of the eyes because there is a direct neurological connection between the eight suboccipital muscles and the muscles that move our eyeballs.

We can directly experience this connection between eye movement and changes in tension of the suboccipital muscles if we place a finger across the back of the head, just under and parallel to the lower edge of the skull. Leaving the head in place, if we move our eyes right or left, up or down, or diagonally, a light finger pressure should detect a slight movement of the upper cervical vertebrae, or a change in the levels of tension in the muscles of the neck under our finger along with every movement of our eyes.

In my clinic I have observed that people who are socially engaged have a well-positioned C1 and C2. They also have a well-functioning autonomic nervous system that is flexible and able to respond appropriately to a variety of situations and internal states.

Social engagement is not a fixed state, nor should the position of C1 and C2 stay fixed after doing the Basic Exercise. These bones move the instant that our psychological state shifts in moments of happiness, satisfaction, fear, anger, or withdrawal, or when our physiological state shifts among social engagement, dorsal vagus activation, or spinal sympathetic chain activation.

Our autonomic nervous system is constantly scanning both our external and internal environments. When everything is good, C1 and C2 come into place, and we get adequate blood flow to the brainstem. When there is a dorsal vagal state, or activity of the spinal sympathetic chain, C1 and C2 rotate out of position, reducing blood flow to the origin of the five cranial nerves in the brainstem and to some areas of the brain. This physiological mechanism takes us away from social engagement, but it also enables us to react when we are challenged or endangered. This mechanism is instinctive, immediate, and bypasses conscious thought. Usually we are not aware of the change.

One of the cornerstones of my treatment of stress and depression is to realign C1 and C2 using the Basic Exercise, or with a hands-on myofascial release technique (see "Neuro-Fascial Release Technique" on page 195). These interventions release imbalances in the tension of the small muscles that hold the skull and the first two vertebrae in relation to each other, and this repositions the atlas and the occiput. Improved alignment of the vertebrae, especially C1 and C2, improves blood flow to the brain and usually brings a rapid improvement in the function of the five nerves necessary for the state of social engagement.

There are other forms of manual therapy that use short-thrust, high-velocity manipulative techniques designed put C1 in place. However, I prefer to use a gentle technique. If I can give the body the right information with a soft touch at the right place, the body will balance itself. Because we cannot put C1 and C2 into place and expect them to stay that way permanently, we should repeat balancing techniques frequently, or as needed. Since there is no such thing as a fixed state of balance, it is more useful to think of *balancing,* an ongoing process.

Neuro-Fascial Release Technique for Social Engagement

Before I ever heard of the Polyvagal Theory or treated a patient on the autism spectrum, I managed to develop a hands-on healing technique on the base of the cranium that I would fortuitously be able to use later to help many people improve their communication and social skills. Sometimes I choose to use this technique in my clinic rather than the Basic Exercise. I've named it the "Neuro-Fascial Release Technique."

I developed this technique based on my understanding of the principles of biomechanical craniosacral therapy, osteopathy, and connective-tissue release (Rolfing). I have used it with great success for at least twenty-five years, and I have taught it to a few thousand therapists.

This technique takes less than five minutes to perform, requires no physical effort, and is highly effective. You can use it on yourself, or to treat someone else.

WHEN TO UTILIZE THE NEURO-FASCIAL RELEASE TECHNIQUE

The Basic Exercise is a simple self-help method, and an easy and effective way to achieve better function of the ventral vagus nerve. However, if you are a body therapist, you may prefer to use your own hands rather than give people exercises to do; or you may want to combine the self-help exercises with hands-on techniques.

The Neuro-Fascial Release Technique can serve as an alternative to the Basic Exercise. It is especially valuable for treating babies, children, and adults on the autism spectrum who lack the necessary verbal communication skills to absorb instruction about the Basic Exercise, when it might be difficult to communicate with them and have them follow your instructions. Using your hands in this way gives you a nonverbal method for bringing about beneficial changes in another person's nervous system.

If you practice massage or other hands-on modalities, I suggest that you do this technique, or have your client do the Basic Exercise, when you start your sessions. This recommendation is in line with the research of Porges, Cottingham, and Lyon (see earlier section), and will ensure that your client's autonomic nervous system will be flexible and that he will gain the most he can from your treatment.

I also suggest that you end your sessions with this technique.

NEURO-FASCIAL RELEASE TECHNIQUE INSTRUCTIONS

If you are used to doing massage, you will need to use your hands in a new way in order to have success with this technique. Practice this technique on yourself and learn how to achieve a release before you try it on someone else. To bring about social engagement with this technique, you need to stimulate reflexes in the nerves in the loose connective tissue just under the skin over the base of the skull. This balances the levels of tension in the small muscles between the base of the skull and the vertebrae of the neck.

It will be easier to learn this technique if the person is lying on his stomach, so that you can easily see your fingers. Start with one side of the back of his head.

1. Push gently at the base of the skull on one side, and feel the hardness of the occipital bone. Test the "slide-ability" of the skin on one side of the occiput. Gently slide the skin over the bone to the right. Then let it come back to neutral.

2. Then slide the skin to the left, and let it come back to neutral. In which direction was there more resistance?

3. Slide the skin in the direction of greater resistance. Go very slowly, and be ready to stop at the very first sign of resistance. It may only have moved an eighth of an inch or less. Stop there, and hold that position. Continue to feel the slight resistance. In the pause when

you are doing nothing, the person will sigh or swallow, and the resistance in the skin will melt away as it releases.

4. When you test again, the skin should slide easily in both directions.

5. Repeat the technique on the other side.

When you test the vagus nerve again (see Chapter 4), it should be functioning properly. Also, there should be greater freedom of movement when turning the head to the left and right.

TWO-HANDED NEURO-FASCIAL RELEASE TECHNIQUE INSTRUCTIONS

Once you have practiced with one hand, you can use two hands.

1. Place one finger of one hand on the occiput at the base of the back of the head on one side. Test the slide-ability of the skin over the bone, as described above. The skin should slide more easily in one direction than the other over the bone.

2. Place a finger from the other hand at the top of the neck on the same side. If you push a little deeper, you should be able to feel the muscles. Use this finger to test the slide-ability of the skin over the muscles at the top of the neck. It should move more easily in the direction opposite to the direction that the other finger is sliding over the skull bone (Figure 9).

3. After you have tested, lighten your pressure. Let the fingers of your two hands slide the skin in opposite directions until you feel resistance.

4. Stop there, and hold that slight tension; wait until you get a sigh or a swallow.

5. Release your fingers, and allow the skin to return to its original position.

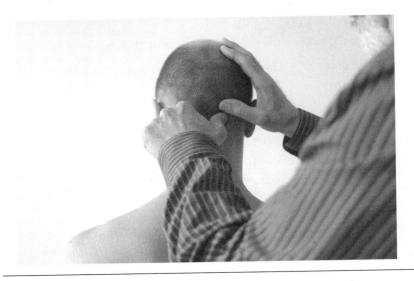

Figure 9. Sliding the skin over the occiput with two hands

6. Do the same thing on the skin on the opposite side of the skull and the neck.

When you test the vagus nerve again, it should now be functioning properly. There should also be greater freedom of movement when turning the head to the left and to the right.

PROPER APPLICATION OF THE NEURO-FASCIAL RELEASE TECHNIQUE

The key to success with the Neuro-Fascial Release Technique is getting the skin to slide, and stopping at the first sign of resistance. Use your fingertips to connect with the skin using the lightest touch imaginable. Then slide the skin a very short distance over the underlying layers of muscles, bones, and tendons.

This technique differs from techniques used in other forms of massage, which primarily target the muscular system and therefore push into the body. Please take the time to read the step-by-step instructions so that you can learn to do it properly.

This hands-on technique stretches the loose connective tissue just under the skin. (To get an appreciation of how fine and delicate this tissue is, go to YouTube and search "Strolling under the Skin.") This connective tissue is rich in proprioceptive nerve endings. When you gently slide the skin a very short distance over the muscles and bones, you create a slight traction in this loose tissue, which is enough to stimulate these nerves.

You slide the skin only a short distance, until you feel the very first sign of resistance, and because you are working directly on the proprioceptive nerves you do not need to use the force required by most forms of massage that focus on the muscles. If you use unnecessary force and keep pushing after the first sign of resistance, or if you slide the skin too rapidly, the muscles and the ligaments will actually tighten. You cannot cause any damage this way—the release just takes a longer time. At worst, you might not get the desired changes.

You may find that sometimes you are pushing so lightly that the other person reports that they cannot feel anything. That is good feedback!

As you progress with the treatment, you will notice palpable improvement in the slide-ability of the skin.

The Salamander Exercises

The following "Salamander Exercises" progressively increase flexibility in the thoracic spine, freeing up movement in the joints between the individual ribs and the sternum. This will increase your breathing capacity, help reduce a forward head posture by bringing your head back into better alignment, and reduce a scoliosis (abnormal spine curvature).

Eighty percent of the fibers of the vagus nerve are afferent (sensory) fibers, which means that they bring information back from the body to the brain, while only 20 percent are efferent (motor) fibers that carry instructions from the brain to the body. Some of the afferent fibers from parts of CN IX and CN X monitor the amount of oxygen and carbon dioxide in the blood. By improving our pattern of breathing with these exercises, we tell the brain (via the afferent nerves) that we are safe and that our visceral organs are functioning properly. This in turn facilitates ventral vagal activity.

But which comes first? Is a limited breathing pattern the result of a dysfunctional ventral vagus, or is a lack of ventral vagus function caused by feedback from a less than optimal breathing pattern? If there are tensions in the respiratory diaphragm and the muscles that move the ribs, feedback from the afferent vagal nerves monitoring those movements will report abnormal breathing, which may prevent a state of ventral vagal activity, just as restoring ventral vagal activity can improve the physiological condition; in practice, improving either one is helpful, no matter which came first.

A forward head posture reduces the space in the upper chest that is available for breathing. The Salamander Exercises can create more space in the upper chest for both the heart and the lungs. Reducing a forward head posture will also take pressure off of the nerves that reach from the spinal cord to the heart, lungs, and visceral organs. By improving the alignment of the cervical vertebrae, the Salamander Exercises also relieve pressure on vertebral arteries, and can relieve some back pains between the shoulders.

When you do the Salamander Exercises, you bring your head to the same level as the rest of your spine. This posture is similar to that of a salamander, which does not have a neck, so that its head is like an extra vertebra at the top of the spine. A salamander cannot flex, extend, rotate, or side-bend its head separately in relationship to the first vertebra of the spine, or lift its head above the level of the spinal vertebrae, as reptiles and mammals can. This exercise is done with the head in line with the spine.

In terms of your spinal movements, these exercises put your head in a position that is neither up nor down. The thoracic (chest portion of the spine) can now side-bend better, somewhat like a salamander. You can utilize side-bending movements in your thoracic vertebrae in order to release muscular tensions between your ribs and thoracic spine. This contributes to the freedom of movement of your ribs and promotes optimal breathing.

In the extension and flexion of the human spine, there is usually greater flexibility in the neck and lumbar vertebrae, and less flexibility in the thoracic spine. However, the flexibility of the thoracic spine increases dramatically with side-bending. The facet joints of the thoracic vertebrae are unlocked, allowing the thoracic spine to side-bend more freely.

LEVEL 1: THE HALF-SALAMANDER EXERCISE

To do the first part of the Salamander Exercise to the right, sit or stand in a comfortable position.

1. Without turning your head, let your eyes look to the right.

2. Continuing to face straight forward, tilt your head to the right so that your right ear moves closer to your right shoulder, without lifting the shoulder to meet it (Figure 10).

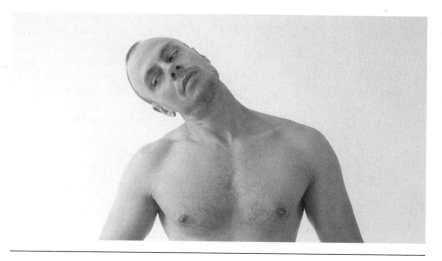

Figure 10. Half-Salamander with eyes to the right

3. Hold your head in this position for thirty to sixty seconds.

4. Then let your head come back up to neutral, and shift your eyes to look forward again.

5. Now do the same on the other side: let your eyes look to the left, and then side-bend your head to the left. After thirty to sixty seconds, return your head to an upright position, and your eyes to a forward direction.

THE HALF-SALAMANDER—A VARIATION

In this variation on the Half-Salamander Exercise, follow the same instructions above, but let your eyes look to the *right* while tipping your head to the *left* (Figure 11). This movement of your eyes in the opposite direction before you move your head increases your range of motion; you should be able to side-bend your head even further to the left. Hold this for thirty to sixty seconds, and then reverse to do the same thing on the other side.

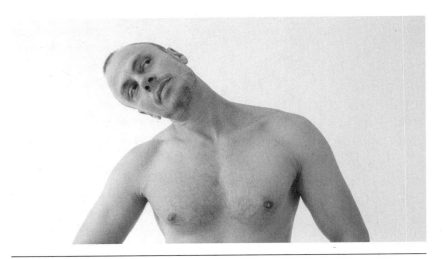

Figure 11. Half-Salamander with eyes to the left

LEVEL 2: THE FULL SALAMANDER EXERCISE

The Full Salamander Exercise involves side-bending the entire spine rather than just the neck. Also, we use a different body position.

1. Get down on all fours, supporting your weight on your knees and the palms of your hands. You can rest your hands on the floor, but it is better if you place the palms of your hands on a desktop, a table, the seat of a chair, or the pillows of a sofa. Your head should be on the same plane as your spine (Figure 12).

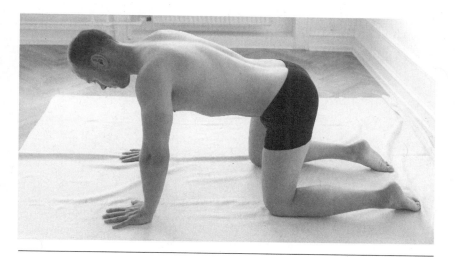

Figure 12. Salamander on all fours

2. In this exercise, your ears should be neither lifted above nor dropped below the level of your spine. In order to find the right head position, lift your head slightly above what you think is right. You should be able to sense that your head is slightly raised. Then lower your head slightly below what you think is right. You should be able to sense that your head is lower than it should be. Go back and forth between the two positions. Take your head up a little and then take it down a little. Try to find a position in the middle where your head does not feel too far up or down. Although you may never find this position exactly, you can begin to zero in on it.

3. Once you have found a good position for your head relative to your spine, look to the right with your eyes, hold them in that position, and side-bend your head to the right by moving your right ear toward your right shoulder.

4. Complete the movement by letting the bend in your side continue beyond your neck, all the way down to the base of your spine.

5. Hold this position for thirty to sixty seconds.

6. Bring your spine and head back to center.

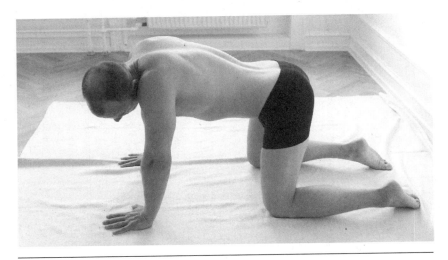

Figure 13. Salamander with head to the left

7. Repeat all steps above, but on the left side (Figure 13).

Massage for Migraines

In the Appendix you will find drawings of four different patterns of migraine headache pain, shown in red. (See "Headache" illustrations.) The X's in the drawings indicate the location of trigger points on the surface of the muscles that can be massaged in order to release tension in the affected muscles.

The four drawings show the four typical patterns of migraine pain. Find the pattern of pain that fits your symptoms. Once you identify the headache pattern, you can see which part of which muscle has been tight, and where to massage it.

The trigger points, each marked with an *X* in each drawing, are areas on the surface of a muscle where there is a high concentration of nerve endings. Some of them will feel more thick or hard than the rest of the muscle. People often find that trigger points that need to be released are painful when pressure is applied.

FINDING AND DEFUSING TENSION IN TRIGGER POINTS

Because you are working on nerves on the surface of the muscle, a light touch is usually sufficient to release the tension in the entire muscle. Rather than massaging the entire muscle, as in ordinary massage, it is usually enough to simply massage the trigger points. You do not need to work hard or press deep into the body.

Massaging trigger points deeply or with a lot of force is usually painful, and can be counterproductive. Under excessive pressure, the body does not feel safe, and the autonomic nervous system is put into a state of sympathetic activation or dorsal vagal withdrawal. This is not harmful, but it is inefficient because it takes time for the body to settle down again.

Make a few small circles on the trigger point. Then stop and wait until you notice a nervous system reaction in the form of a sigh or a swallow. Within a few minutes, the intensity of the pain should start to diminish or disappear. You can repeat the treatment whenever relief from a migraine is needed.

Not all the *X*'s on the drawing need to be treated. Even if an *X* indicates a trigger point for a particular pattern of pain, if you do not feel anything hard or painful at that particular spot on the surface of the muscle, that trigger point is not active. Don't waste time trying to release it, but focus on the trigger points that do feel hard, thick, or painful.

SCM Exercise for a Stiff Neck

This exercise will extend your range of movement as you rotate your head, alleviate symptoms of a stiff neck, and help to prevent migraine headaches. It is similar to the very first movements that we made as infants lying on our stomachs, propped up on our elbows, with our heads free to move so that we could look around.

1. Lie on your stomach (Figure 14). Lift your head, and bring your arms under your chest. Rest the weight of your upper body on your elbows (Figure 15).

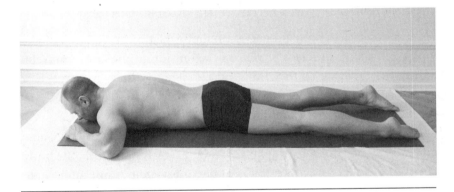

Figure 14. Lying on the stomach

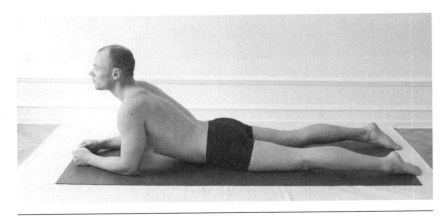

Figure 15. Lifting the head

2. Rotate your head to the right as far as it comfortably goes. Hold that position for sixty seconds.

3. Bring your head back to center.

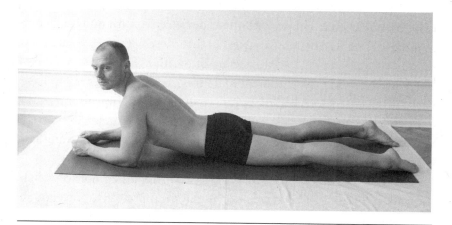

Figure 16. Turning the head to the left

4. Now rotate your head to the left as far as it comfortably goes, and hold that position for sixty seconds (Figure 16).

If you have improved the rotation of the head with this exercise but the movement is still not as good as you want it to be on one side, then the restriction is probably coming from another muscle, the *levator scapulae*, which is innervated by spinal nerves C3–C5. This kind of stiff neck will not be eliminated solely by improving the function of CN XI and the trapezius and sternocleidomastoid muscles. (See "The *Levator Scapulae* Muscle" on page 104).

Part of the stiffness may also come from a hiatal hernia and shortening of the esophagus, since the vagus nerve wraps around the esophagus. (See "Relieving COPD and Hiatal Hernia" on page 91.)

Twist and Turn Exercise for the Trapezius

The Twist and Turn Exercise improves the tone of a flaccid trapezius muscle, and balances each of its three parts with the other two parts. It also helps to lengthen the spine, improve breathing, and correct forward head posture (FHP). This in turn often alleviates shoulder and back pain.

This exercise can benefit anyone, not just those with FHP. It takes less than one minute to do, and the feeling of positive change is immediate. It is a good idea to take a moment to do this exercise whenever you have been sitting for a while, and to repeat it regularly from time to time. I do it almost every time that I get up from sitting at my computer. Every time you do the exercise, you will experience an improvement in breathing and posture, and its positive effects are cumulative.

The idea behind this exercise is neither to strengthen nor to stretch the trapezius muscle. The assumption is that the muscle is strong enough and just needs stimulation of the nerves to flaccid muscle fibers. You are waking them up so that they can take over their share of the work, as they did when we were babies and crawled on all fours.

When a baby is lying on its stomach, it uses all the fibers of the three parts of the trapezius muscle to keep the shoulder blades together, lift the head, and turn the head to look around. Later, the baby also uses all these muscle fibers when raising itself up on all fours to crawl and to look around.

However, when a baby stands up, all the fibers of the trapezius are no longer used evenly. Some become more tense, while the energy goes out of other fibers so that they become flaccid. The head is no longer supported in the same way by all three parts of the trapezius muscle. Over time, the head tends to glide further forward, so that the centers of the ears are in front of the center of the shoulders. The shoulders then exhibit a tendency to pull forward and down toward the midline.

After doing this exercise, you will have a more even tone in all the muscle fibers of the three parts of your trapezius. Then, when you stand or sit, your head will glide back and up naturally by itself, reducing FHP and improving your posture.

TWIST AND TURN EXERCISE INSTRUCTIONS

There are three parts to this exercise. The difference between the three parts is the position of your arms.

1. Sit comfortably on a firm surface, such as the seat of a chair or a bench. Keep your face looking forward.

2. Fold and cross your arms, with your hands resting lightly on your elbows (Figure 17). You will be rotating your shoulder girdle briskly, first to one side and then to the other, without stopping, and without shifting the hips.

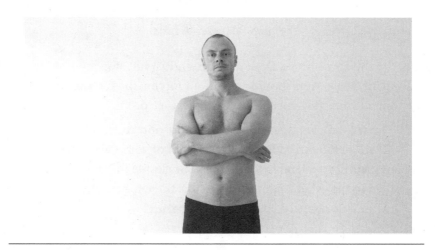

Figure 17. Hands on elbows

3. For the first part of the exercise, let your elbows drop and rest just in front of your body. Rotate your shoulders so that your elbows move, first to one side and then back to the other side. When you rotate your shoulders from side to side, your arms glide lightly over your stomach. This activates the fibers of your upper trapezius (Figure 18).

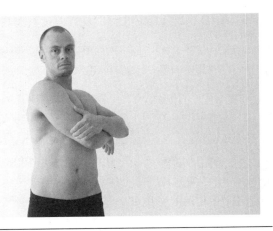

Figure 18. Trapezius twist

4. Do this three times. Do not strain, and do not stop your movement. Move your shoulders without forcing them or holding them; your movements are easy and relaxed.

5. The second part is just like the first; the only difference is that you lift your elbows and hold them in front of your chest, at the level of your heart (Figure 19). Rotate your elbows first to one side and then to the other (Figure 20). Do this three times. This activates the muscle fibers of your middle trapezius.

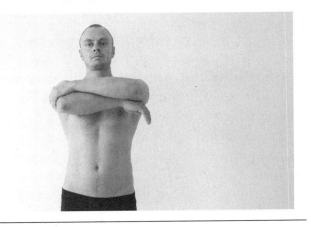

Figure 19. Trapezius twist with elbows lifted

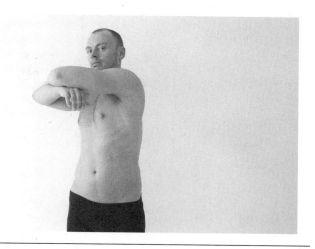

Figure 20. Trapezius twist to the right

6. For the third part, raise your elbows as high as you comfortably can, and repeat the exercise above (Figure 21). Rotate your elbows from side to side, three times (Figure 22). This activates the muscle fibers of your lower trapezius.

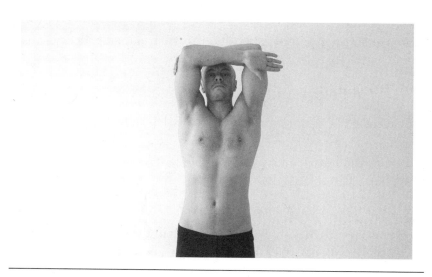

Figure 21. Elbows raised high

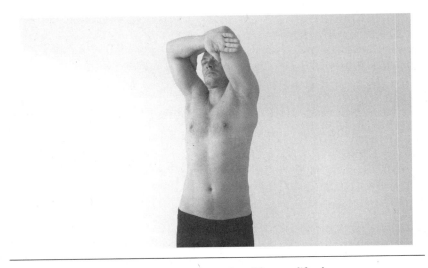

Figure 22. Trapezius twist with arms lifted

After you have done the exercise, you might notice that your head feels lighter and has moved back and up, away from the forward head posture. It is not uncommon for someone with significant FHP to become an inch or two taller the first time they do the exercise. If someone has been looking at you from the side, she will see that your head has moved partway back from its original forward position, if you had that tendency.

A Four-Minute Natural Facelift, Part 1

Benefits of this gentle and pleasant treatment include relaxing the facial muscles and leaving a more natural smile in place by improving the function of cranial nerves V and VII. You can do it for yourself and share it with others. This exercise:

- improves the circulation to your skin
- puts life into the muscles of expression of the middle third of your face, in the area between the corners of the mouth and the corners of the eyes

- improves blood circulation to the skin of your face
- brings a youthful quality of liveliness that you can feel and others can see
- helps you smile more naturally and more often
- makes your face more responsive to interactions with others, and thereby increases your sense of empathy
- makes flat cheekbones a little more prominent and makes very high cheeks a little flatter.

Before you do this technique, look at your face in a mirror. If you are doing the technique on someone else, give him a hand-held mirror so he can watch his face and follow the changes. Look especially at the area of the skin around the cheekbones.

Do one side of the face first. Then check whether you can see or feel a difference between the two sides. The differences are usually obvious when you talk or smile. Then do the other side. There should be more symmetry again.

WHERE TO DO THE TECHNIQUE

There is a point on the face that is the endpoint of the Large Intestine acupuncture meridian, called LI 20. (See "Acupuncture points" in the Appendix.) It is a beauty point in Chinese, Japanese, and Thai Massage. In Classical Thai Massage, this point is called "Golden Bamboo." In Traditional Chinese Medicine, this point is called "Welcoming Fragrance," and it opens the nostrils, improving the breathing.

This point in Chinese medicine is interesting in terms of Western anatomy. It lies directly over a joint between two bones of the face, the maxilla and the pre-maxilla. The two bones were separate entities long ago in the evolutionary development of our species, but they calcified together into a single bone at an early stage. In modern anatomy, the maxilla/pre-maxilla is referred to as one bone, called the maxilla.

The endpoint of the Large Intestine meridian is easy to find. Just lightly touch the skin about an eighth of an inch to the side of the top of the supra-alar crease (the fold between the cheek and upper lip), near the outer edge of the nostril. If you explore the area with your finger, you will find this point easily because it is more sensitive than the rest of the surrounding skin (Figure 23).

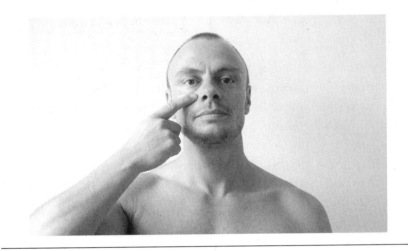

Figure 23. Massage at LI 20

HOW AND WHY TO DO THE TECHNIQUE

The surface of the facial skin is innervated by branches of the fifth cranial nerve. Lightly touching the skin of your face stimulates these nerve endings.

1. With a very light contact, brush the surface of the skin at acupuncture point LI 20. Then let your fingertip melt together with the skin.

2. Slide the skin up and down to find which direction presents greater resistance. Push lightly into that resistance. Stop.

3. Hold at that point, and wait to feel it release.

4. Slide the skin inward toward the midline of the face, and out toward the side to find the direction of greater resistance.

5. Stop there, and push lightly. Hold and wait for the release.

The muscles of the face are innervated by branches of the seventh cranial nerve (VII). There are two layers of facial muscles just below the skin.

6. Let your fingertip sink gently into the muscle layers beneath the skin at the same point. Let the first muscle layer adhere to your fingertip as if it were Velcro.

7. If you are careful not to push too hard, and if you feel what is happening under your fingertips, you can slide these layers of muscles; first slide one layer on top of the other, making a small circle.

8. As you go around the circle, you may notice that there is more resistance to sliding the skin in one direction. Keep pushing lightly in that direction, and hold until there is a release in the form of a sigh or a swallow.

9. Next, push slightly deeper. Now the deeper layer of muscles sticks together with the top muscle layer and the skin. You can slide both layers together over the surface of the bone.

10. As you go around the circle, you may notice that there is more resistance to sliding the skin in one direction. Keep pushing lightly in that direction, and hold until there is a release in the form of a sigh or a swallow.

All bones have a connective-tissue covering called a periosteum (*peri-* means "around," and *osteum* means "bone"). This tissue is very rich in nerve endings from spinal nerves or, in this case, cranial nerves.

11. Let your fingertip sink even deeper into the face until you rest lightly on the surface of the bone.

12. Massage on the surface of the periosteum has a profound effect on the autonomic nervous system. Press lightly, but hard enough

to reach the surface of the bone at Large Intestine 20. Let your fingertip move from side to side on the surface of the bone, then hold a light pressure on the bone and wait until you get a release.

In the embryo, this bone was two bones, the maxilla and the pre-maxilla. Even though these have fused into one bone, it is still possible for most people to sense that there were once two separate bones.

This massage of cranial nerves V and VII stimulates the nerves to the skin and muscles of the face. It does not erase all the wrinkles, but it relaxes the muscles of the face, reduces some wrinkles, and leaves the face looking younger and more refreshed. And there are no negative side-effects such as scar tissue from a face-lift operation or toxic accumulations of Botox.

More importantly, this massage helps the face to be more expressive, communicative, and responsive—more socially engaged. Our face should be flexible and able to express different emotional responses in various situations. Facial expressions are a vital part of our communication with other people.

In addition to expressing our own emotions, facial flexibility is impor-tant for social engagement. When our face is relaxed and we look at some-one else's face, our own face automatically makes micro-movements that mirror the other's facial expression. These movements are very small, and change very quickly.

These changes in tension in our skin and our facial muscles then feed back to the brain via the afferent pathways of cranial nerves V and VII, to give us immediate subconscious information about what others are feeling. This is a prerequisite for us to have empathy for another person.

If facial muscles under the skin are generally relaxed, a person usually has a smooth, pleasant, and what is seen as a beautiful or handsome face. Unfortunately, many people get stuck in the same emotional and facial pattern for years. Their facial muscles pull on the skin, creating wrinkles or a double chin. If the person stays in the same emotional state and does not relax his or her facial muscles, these wrinkles become deeper with time.

In addition to this technique, a light stroking of the skin of the face stimulates CN V and reduces tension in all the facial muscles.

A Four-Minute Natural Facelift, Part 2

Part 1 is focused on LI20, an acupuncture point on the Large Intestine meridian at the side of the nostril. Stimulating this point improves the balance and tone of the muscles of the lower face around the mouth and the nose. Part 2, in turn, focuses on the eyes. The actual technique is similar in many ways to the first facelifting technique that you did at Large Intestine 20. You will find acupuncture point B2 on the inside corner of the eyebrow. People often rub this point naturally, without thinking about it, when they are tired. Massaging the skin and muscles of the face here is often self-soothing (Figure 24).

Using your thumb or one finger, connect to B2. At B2, work your way down each of the layers: the skin, two layers of muscles, and the periosteum.

This point is also a trigger point for the orbicularis oculi muscle, a thin, flat muscle that surrounds the opening of the eye. The eyes are

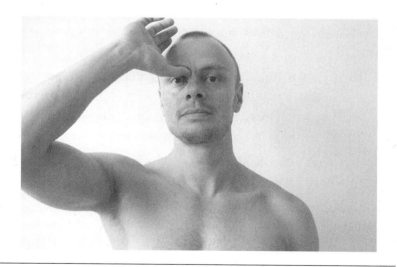

Figure 24. Massage at B2

sometimes called the mirror of the soul. Before we work on B2, the muscle might be too tight, leaving the eye somewhat closed or it might be under-toned, leaving the eye too open. When we finish, there will be an improved balance between looking outwards and looking in. You will see another person more clearly, and this person in turn will have an easier time making eye contact with you and will experience seeing you differently .

At a deeper level, this acupuncture point is at the edge of a tiny facial bone called the lacrimal bone. The word "lacrimal" refers to tears. Some-times a person's eyes can be dry and appear lifeless. Someone can also experience an annoying flow of tears

By touching this bone at B2 and holding your contact on the lacrimal bone, you will balance the flow of moisture to the eyes and leave them bright and sparkling. The goal of the facelifting massage is leave a smile on your lips and a twinkle in your eyes.

1. Find the place at the inner corner of the eyebrow that is more sensitive than the surrounding areas.

2. First use your fingertip to brush the skin lightly a few times.

3. Let your fingertip rest lightly on the skin at point B2 (see above), and hold that contact with the surface of the skin until you get a release in the form of sigh or a swallow.

4. Next, press gently down to the layer of the facial muscles. This is where the flat, round *orbicularis oculi* muscle, which goes around the eye, attaches to the bones of the face. Let the skin stick to your finger and make a small circle, sliding the skin lightly and searching for the direction where there is resistance.

5. Hold your finger on that resistance until you get a release in the form of a sigh or a swallow.

6. Then go even deeper until you feel the surface of the bone. Rub that a few times.

7. Then hold the contact with the bone, and wait for a release.

If the *orbicularis oculi* muscle is too tight, closing the eyelids into a squint, this should open the eye more normally. If the eye was too wide-open, this technique should firm it down a bit but still leave it open.

This is the second of two beauty points in Classical Thai Massage.

Severing all the Heads of the Hydra

The purpose of all of these self-help exercises and hands-on techniques is to help bring people out of a dorsal vagal state, or help them out of chronic activation of the sympathetic chain, and bring them home to a ventral vagal state. Only in this way can we sever all the heads of the Hydra and restore our capability for physical and emotional health.

Appendix

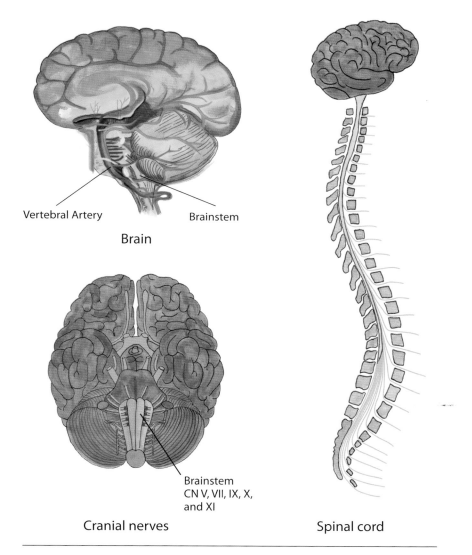

Vertebral Artery

Brainstem

Brain

Brainstem
CN V, VII, IX, X,
and XI

Cranial nerves

Spinal cord

The brainstem extends from the brain; it lies on the underside of the brain and is the beginning of the spinal cord. Cranial nerves, except for cranial nerves I (olfactory) and II (optic), originate in the brainstem. The vertebral artery supplies blood to the brainstem and the five cranial nerves.

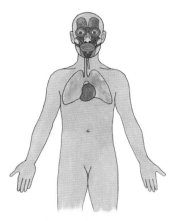

Ventral vagus

The two divisions of the vagus nerve each go to the heart, the lungs, and the airways. In addition to this, the ventral vagus branch extends to the muscles of the throat (larynx and pharynx), and it relates to movements of the face. In the drawing, the red represents the heart, and the blue represents the lungs and the two tubes—the bronchial on the left and the esophagus on the right.

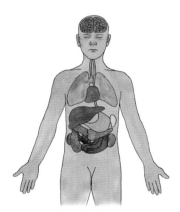

Dorsal vagus

In addition to reaching the heart and lungs, the dorsal vagus nerve branch goes to the subdiaphragmatic organs of digestion (except for the descending colon). It goes to the stomach, liver, pancreas, spleen, ascending colon, and transverse colon. In the drawing, blue stands for the lungs, red for the heart, green for the stomach, brown for the liver, grey-green for the pancreas, darker blue for the ascending and transverse parts of the large intestine, yellow for the spleen, and grey for the small intestine.

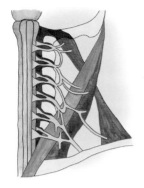 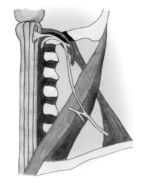 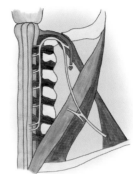

CN XI

These illustrations show the different branches of CN XI. The drawing on the left shows branches which originate in the spinal cord at the level of the cervical vertebrae and go directly to the trapezius and the sternocleidomastoid muscles. The middle drawing shows branches that originate in the spinal cord at the level of the cervical vertebrae and go up into the skull and then exit the skull through the jugular foramen and go to the two muscles. In the drawing on the right, the branch originates in the brain stem, exits the skull through the jugular foramen, and then goes to the two muscles. All of these nerves going to different bundles of muscle fibers allow flexibility and precision in the movement of the neck.

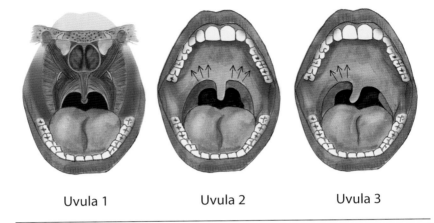

| Uvula 1 | Uvula 2 | Uvula 3 |

To test the pharyngeal branch of the ventral vagus nerve branch: The *levator veli pala-*
tini muscle should pull the soft palate up when we say "ah, ah, ah" in a percussive
manner. The uvula should go up symmetrically, as in "Uvula 2." If it goes up to one
side but not the other, as in "Uvula 3," then there is a dysfunction of the pharyngeal
branch of the ventral vagus on the side that doesn't rise equally.

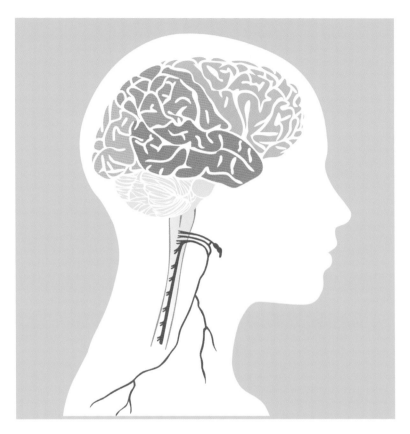

Central nervous system

In this illustration you can see a representation of the central nervous system, showing the brain, the brainstem (a narrowing of the lower part of the brain, which continues down into the body as the spinal cord), and one of the five cranial nerves that has its origin in the brain stem.

All of the twelve cranial nerves originate on the inferior (bottom) surface of the brain or from the brainstem. We are especially interested in CN V, VII, IX, X, and XI. All five of these nerves need to function properly if we are to be socially engaged. In order to function properly, these cranial nerves need an adequate blood supply. Rotation of the atlas, axis, or other cervical vertebrae can reduce the blood supply to the brainstem, resulting in dysfunction in these cranial nerves.

The eleventh cranial nerve (CN XI), one of the five nerves necessary for social engagement, also innervates the trapezius and sternocleidomastoid muscles.

Trapezius

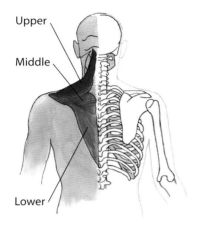

Upper

Middle

Lower

The trapezius muscle has three parts: the upper (in the illustration, dark red), middle (red), and lower (purple).

Sternocleidomastoid

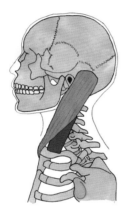

Here you can see a drawing of the sternocleidomastoid muscle. The sternocleidomastoid muscles, one on either side, allow us to turn our head to the right or left. Working together, the trapezius and sternocleidomastoid muscles allow us to move our head precisely, to position our eyes, ears, and nostrils to get important information from our environment.

Supraspinatus

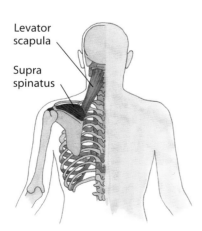

Levator scapula

Supra spinatus

The supraspinatus muscle runs along the top of the shoulder blade.

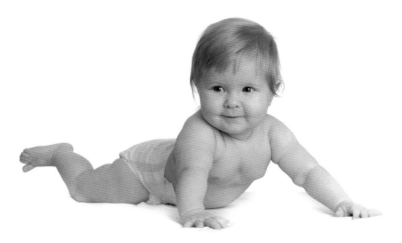

Baby on stomach

When a baby is lying on its stomach, one of the first movements it makes is to lift its head. To do this, it tenses all three parts of its trapezius muscle. Tightening the fibers of its upper trapezius tips its head back and up. Tightening its middle trapezius pulls its shoulder blades together and stabilizes its arms so that they can support the weight of its body. Tightening the lower trapezius allows it to arch the entire length of the spine.

In the photo, you can see that the head is lifted up and tipped back. The shoulder blades are pulled together in the back. The entire length of the spine is arched in a bow. Then, when, the baby has lifted its head, it adds the sternocleidomastoid muscles' activity to rotate its head. The combined action of the trapezius and the sternocleidomastoid muscles allows it to move its head and focus its senses of sight, smell, and hearing on objects of interest anywhere in front of it.

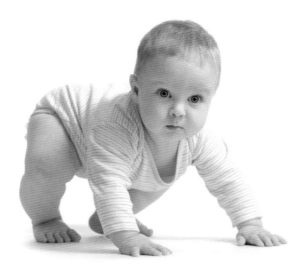

Baby on all fours

When the baby comes up on its hands and feet to crawl, the three parts of the upper, middle, and lower trapezius muscles continue to tighten in the same way as when it lay on its stomach and lifted its head.

However, this relationship changes drastically when the baby stands up on its legs. The upper trapezius no longer tips its head up and back as it did when the baby crawled on all fours.

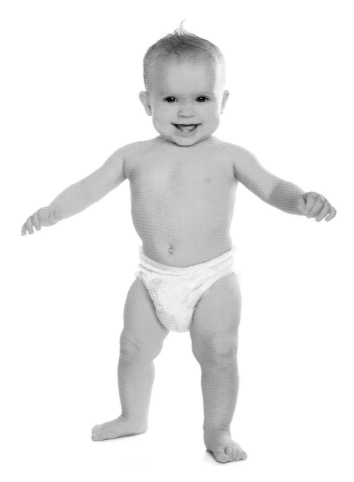

Baby standing

If the relationship between the head and the body were the same as when crawling on all fours, the head would be rotated ninety degrees, with the face looking straight up towards the sky. However, when standing, the head rotates to face forward. Therefore, the upper trapezius has much less tension in a standing position compared with lying on the stomach or crawling on all fours. A forward head posture comes from an upper trapezius that is not too tight but too flaccid. As years pass, the upper trapezius becomes even more and more slack, and the head slides increasingly forward on C1.

The Twist and Turn trapezius exercise in Part Two of this book helps to bring the head back into better alignment because it stimulates all three parts of the muscle.

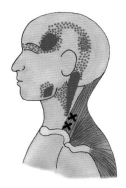

Headache 1

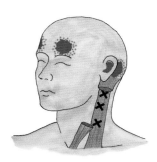

Headache 2

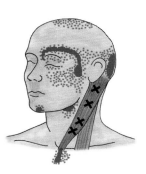

Headache 3

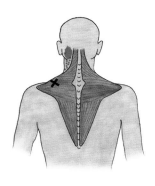

Headache 4

Based on years of experience in my private clinic, and contrary to widely accepted medical practice, I believe that dysfunction of CN XI, which innervates the trapezius and SCM muscles, is involved in migraine headaches.

Migraine headaches are tension headaches, and there are four kinds, each caused by a different pattern of tension in either the sternocleidomastoid or trapezius muscles. If you are having a migraine, look at the four drawings and see if you recognize which pattern of pain (in red) has been plaguing you.

Because these parts of the muscles are innervated by CN XI, the first step in treatment of migraines is to establish proper function of CN XI using the Basic Exercise (see Part Two). Then find the appropriate trigger points (TP), each marked by an *X*, and massage these for a few minutes until you feel relief.

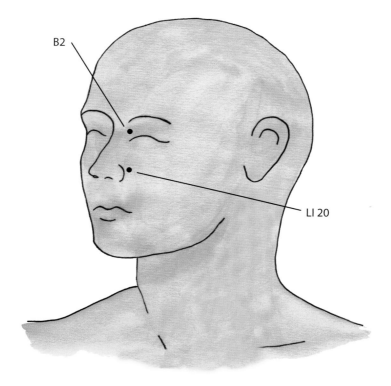

B2

LI 20

Acupuncture points

Massage of acupuncture points for the Natural Facelift for CN V and CN VII: LI 20 (the acupuncture point Large Intestine of the top of the nostril on each side), and B2 (at the inside of the eyebrow).

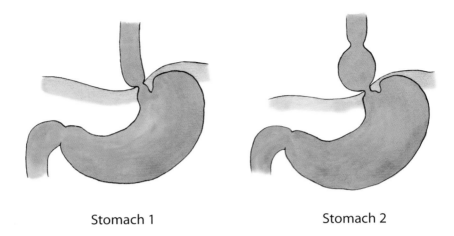

Stomach 1   Stomach 2

Normally, the stomach should be down in the abdomen, well below the respiratory diaphragm. The esophagus is a muscular tube running from the pharynx (back of the throat) into the stomach, passing through an opening (hiatus) in the respiratory diaphragm and into the stomach. When we swallow, the esophagus carries food from the throat to the stomach.

"Stomach 2" shows a hiatal hernia. The upper third of the esophagus is innervated by the ventral vagus nerve. If there is ventral vagus dysfunction, the esophagus shortens, pulling the stomach up against the bottom of the diaphragm and creating a hiatal hernia. Part of the stomach may even be pulled up into the thoracic cavity. This disturbs the proper function of the diaphragm, which cannot descend as it should on the inbreath.

I have found a dorsal vagal state together with a hiatal hernia in almost everyone who has come to my clinic with a diagnosis of COPD.

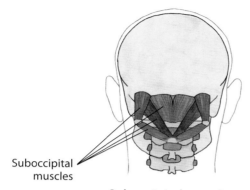

Suboccipital
muscles

Suboccipital muscles

The four pairs of suboccipital muscles are located below the occipital bone at the base of the skull. The suboccipital triangle is a region of the neck bounded by three of these muscle pairs: the *rectus capitis posterior major* (above and medial); the *obliquus capitis superior* (above and lateral); and the *obliquus capitis inferior* (below and lateral).

Whereas the trapezius and sternocleidomastoid muscles are responsible for the gross movements of the head on the neck, the suboccipital muscles allow for finer control of these movements.

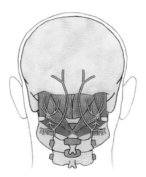

Suboccipital nerve

The suboccipital muscles are innervated by the suboccipital nerve, which passes through the suboccipital triangle and branches to the suboccipital muscles.

Using the gentle techniques in the Basic Exercise, we can balance the tensions in these muscles. Then the bones can assume a better position with regard to each other, allowing more blood to flow through the vertebral arteries. There is often an almost instantaneous improvement of not only the position of the bones but also the function of the ventral vagus nerve branch.

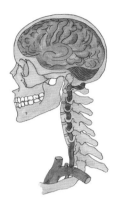

Vertebral arteries

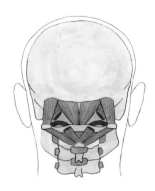

Suboccipal muscles
with vertebra

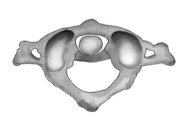

Atlas

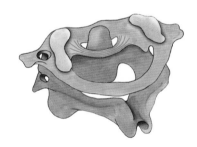

Axis and atlas

The suboccipital muscles play a critical role in stabilizing the head on the neck by stabilizing the cranium on the atlas (the top neck vertebra, or C1) and the atlas on the axis (the second vertebra, C2).

Tensions in the muscles of the suboccipital triangle can pull the occiput, C1, and C2 away from their optimal position in relationship to each other. Tightening and imbalance of the suboccipital muscles can also put pressure on the nerves and blood vessels in the suboccipital triangle.

The vertebral artery (red) passes between the suboccipital muscles on its way to the brainstem, so tension in these muscles can also reduce blood flow to the brainstem.

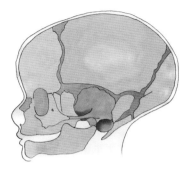

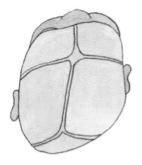

Baby cranium   Baby cranium from above

A flat back of the head is caused by chronic tension in the sternocleidomastoid muscle on one side of the head—most often the right side. This tension is most likely caused by a dysfunction in CN XI.

There are eight bones in the cranium, and fourteen in the face. At birth, the bones have not yet calcified and grown together at the sutures. They are joined by tough sheets of elastic connective tissue. The flexibility of these bones, and the elasticity of the connective tissue between them, are important in the birthing process. The cranium is compressed under tremendous pressure as it travels down the birth canal, and it is not a straight passage. The cranium's flexibility allows it to change shape as it passes through this irregularly shaped tube.

After birth, muscles of the neck and the forces of the fluids inside the cranium begin to bring the baby's head into a more symmetrical and rounded form. A chronic pulling from the sternocleidomastoid muscle, however, is enough to pull the individual bones of the skull out of shape in relationship to each other.

A change in the shape of the back of the head can affect the blood supply to the brain—some parts get an excessive blood supply, and other parts a reduced supply. Since I have become aware of the shape of the back of the head, I have noticed a flat back of the head on every one of my clients on the autistic spectrum or with ADHD. The drawing "Baby cranium from above" illustrates a severe case of deformation of the cranium, usually caused by a tight sternocleidomastoid muscle.

It is possible to lessen skull deformation by releasing chronic tension in the SCM muscle on one side, even in adults in whom the bones of the skull are believed to have grown together so that the shape of the skull is fixed. Far from it! It is surprising how much you can round a flattened back of the head, regardless of age.

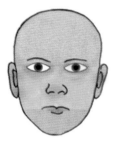

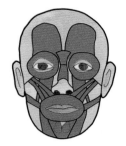

Face   Facial muscles

Many of us do not have much movement in the muscles of our face. Face-muscle movement can occur spontaneously, or can be consciously put on, such as, for example, when we smile for a photo.

Spontaneous changes of facial expression, especially when someone is looking directly at another person, are a sign of social engagement. These small changes occur at a rate of several times per second. The individual expressions are too fast to notice, but we can see that there is life in the face.

When someone is socially engaged, the spontaneous facial movements occur in the zone between a line drawn across the middle part of the eyes and a line between her lips.

NOTES

1 Jerzy Grotowski, ed. Eugenio Barba, *Towards a Poor Theatre* (New York: Routledge Theatre Arts, 2002), 27.

2 Ida P. Rolf, PhD, *Rolfing: Reestablishing the Natural Alignment and Structural Integration of the Human Body for Vitality and Well-Being,* rev. ed. (Rochester, VT: Healing Arts Press, 1989).

3 "The Nobel Prize in Physiology or Medicine 1937," *Nobel Media AB 2014* (Oct 4, 2016), www.nobelprize.org/nobel_prizes/medicine /laureates/1937/.

4 There is another aspect and medical definition of stress that refers to pushing our muscles and/or organs with sports training and other physical regimens such as fasting, and it has been said that a certain level of this kind of stress is good for an organism.

5 Alain Gehin's definitive book on his technique is called *The Atlas of Manipulative Techniques for the Cranium and the Face* (Seattle: Eastland Press, English translation, 1985). In this book, Gehin teaches more than 150 biomechanical techniques, and describes which techniques to choose when attempting to improve the function of the individual cranial nerves.

6 Ronald Lawrence and Stanley Rosenberg, *Pain Relief with Osteomassage* (Santa Barbara, CA: Woodbridge Press, 1982).

7 CN VIII is the coccleovestibular nerve. There are two specialized organs in the bony labyrinth of the temporal bone. "Cochlear" refers to the auditory component of CN VIII, which transduces sound into electrical impulses to the brain. "Vestibular" refers to the part of CN VIII that translates information from the movement of a thick fluid in three semicircular canals embedded in the temporal bone. As we change the position of the head in relationship to gravity, fluid in these canals moves, pushing on hairs that stimulate nerves to give us information about the position and movement of the head.

8 Harold Magoun, DO, *Osteopathy in the Cranial Field,* 3rd ed. (India-napolis, IN: The Cranial Academy, 1976).

9 The idea that the cranial bones move is contrary to almost all teachings in anatomy and physiology. The commonly held belief is that the bones fuse together at different ages, the last of these growing fast to the rest of the skull at the age of thirty-eight. However, I saw collections of separate human skull bones from an older adult in an anatomy lab; the bones had been separated by filling a prepared skull with rice and submerging it in a bucket of water. As the rice absorbed the water and expanded, it pushed the bones apart from each other. If the bones had fully grown together, as is taught in many anatomy classes, this separation of bones would not be possible in an adult of this age.

10 Lauren M. Wier, MPH (Thomson Reuters) and Roxanne M. Andrews, PhD (AHRQ), *Statistical Brief #107: The National Hospital Bill: The Most Expensive Conditions by Payer, 2008*, Healthcare Cost and Utilization Project Statistical Brief #107 (Rockville, MD: Agency for Healthcare Research and Quality, 2011), www.hcup-us.ahrq.gov/reports /statbriefs/sb107.pdf.

11 M. Widen, "Back Specialists are Discouraging the Use of Surgery," American Academy of Pain Medicine, 17th annual meeting, Miami Beach, FL (2001).

12 Markus Melloh, Christoph Röder, Achim Elfering, Jean-Claude Theis, Urs Müller, Lukas P. Staub, Emin Aghayev, Thomas Zweig, Thomas Barz, Thomas Kohlmann, Simon Wieser, Peter Jüni, and Marcel Zwahlen, "Differences Across Health Care Systems in Outcome and Cost-Utility of Surgical and Conservative Treatment of Chronic Low Back Pain: A Study Protocol," *BMC Musculoskeletal Disorders* 9, no. 81 (2008).

13 *Lumbar Spinal Stenosis*, American Academy of Orthopaedic Surgeons (2010), www.knowyourback.org/Pages/SpinalConditions /DegenerativeConditions/LumbarSpinalStenosis.aspx.

14 Michael Gershon, *The Second Brain* (New York: Harper Collins Publishers, 1999).

15 B. Zahorska-Markiewicz, E. Kuagowska, C. Kucio, and M. Klin, "Heart Rate Variability in Obesity," *International Journal of Obesity and Related Metabolic Disorders* 17, no. 1 (Jan 1993): 21–23.

16 Gernot Ernst, *Heart Rate Variability* (London: Springer-Verlag, 2014), 261.

17 Stephen W. Porges, "Orienting in a Defensive World: Mammalian Modifications of our Evolutionary Heritage—A Polyvagal Theory," *Psychophysiology* 32 (1995): 301–18.

18 Fischer, Philip, MD, "Postural Orthostatic Tachycardia Syndrome (POTS)," Mayo Clinic podcast (Apr 23, 2008), http://newsnetwork .mayoclinic.org/discussion/postural-orthostatic-tachycardia -syndrome-pots-24cc80/.

19 P. J. Carek, S.E. Laibstain, and S.M. Carek, "Exercise for the Treatment of Depression and Anxiety," *The International Journal of Psychiatry in Medicine* 41, no. 1 (2011): 15–28.

20 For a list of health issues that can develop, at least in part, from a dysfunctional ventral branch of the vagus nerve, see the table at the beginning of Part One listing the "Heads of the Hydra."

21 Stephen W. Porges, "Neuroception: A Subconscious System for Detecting Threats and Safety," *Zero to Three* 24, no. 5 (May 2004): 19–24.

22 Ben Hogan, *Five Lessons: The Modern Fundamentals of Golf* (New York: Simon and Schuster, 1957).

23 Vasilios Papaioannou, Ioannis Pneumatikos, and Nikos Maglaveras, "Association of Heart Rate Variability and Inflammatory Response in Patients with Cardiovascular Diseases: Current Strengths and Limitations," *Psychosomatic Medicine* 67, suppl. 1 (2005): S29–S33.

24 B. Pomeranz, R. J. Macauley, M. A. Caudill, I. Kutz, D. Adam, and D. Gordon, "Assessment of Autonomic Function in Humans by Heart Rate Spectral Analysis," *American Journal of Physiology* 248 (1985): H151–H153.

25 U. I. Zulfiqar, D. A. Jurivich, W. Gao, and D. H. Singer, "Relation of High Heart Rate Variability to Healthy Longevity," *American Journal of Cardiology* 105, no. 8 (Apr 15, 2010): 1181–85, doi: 10.1016/j.amj -card.2009.12.022 (epub Feb 20, 2010), erratum 106, no. 1 (Jul 1, 2010): 142.

26 P. Jönsson, "Respiratory Sinus Arrhythmia as a Function of State Anxiety in Healthy Individuals," *International Journal of Psychophysiology* 63 (2007): 48–54.

27 P. Nickel and F. Nachreiner, "Sensitivity and Diagnosticity of the 0.1-Hz Component of Heart Rate Variability as an Indicator of Mental Workload," *Human Factors* 45, no. 4 (2003): 575–90.

28 J. F. Brosschot, E. Van Dijk, and J. F. Thayer, "Daily Worry is Related to Low Heart Rate Variability During Waking and the Subsequent Nocturnal Sleep Period," *International Journal of Psychophysiology* 63 (2007): 39–47.

29 A. J. Camm, M. Malik, J. T. Bigger, G. Breithardt, S. Cerutti, R. J. Cohen, P. Coumel, E .L. Fallen, H. L. Kennedy, R. E. Kleiger, F. Lombardi, A. Malliani, A. J. Moss, J. N. Rottman, G. Schmidt, P. J. Schwartz, and D. H. Singer (Task Force of the European Society of Cardiology and the North American Society of Electrophysiology), "Heart Rate Variability: Standards of Measurement, Physiological Interpretation, and Clinical Use," *Circulation* 93 (1996): 1043–65.

30 Arpi Minassian, PhD, Mark A. Geyer, PhD, Dewleen G. Baker, MD, Caroline M. Nievergelt, PhD, Daniel T. O'Connor, MD, Victoria B. Risbrough, PhD, and the Marine Resiliency Study Team, "Heart Rate Variability in a Large Group of Active-Duty Marines and Relationship to Posttraumatic Stress," *Psychosomatic Medicine* 76, no. 4 (May 2014): 292–301.

31 Vasilios Papaioannou, Ioannis Pneumatikos, and Nikos Maglaveras, "Association of Heart Rate Variability and Inflammatory Response in Patients with Cardiovascular Diseases: Current Strengths and Limitations," *Psychosomatic Medicine* 67, suppl. 1 (2005): S29–S33.

32 Masari Amano, Tomo Kando, U. E. Hidetoshi, and Toshio Moriani, "Exercise Training and Autonomic Nervous System Activity in Obese Individuals," *Medicine and Science in Sports and Exercise* 33 (2001): 1287–91.

33 Amelia M. Stanton, Tierney A. Lorenz, Carey S. Pulverman, and Cindy M. Meston, "Heart Rate Variability: A Risk Factor for Female Sexual Dysfunction," *Applied Psychophysiology and Biofeedback* 40 (2015): 229–37.

34 Ji Yong Lee, Kwan-Joong Joo, Jin Tae Kim, Sung Tae Cho, Dae Sung Cho, Yong-Yeun Won, and Jong Bo Choi, "Heart Rate Variability in Men with Erectile Dysfunction," *International Neurourology Journal* 15, no. 2 (Jun 2011): 87–91.

35 Jacqueline M. Dekker, PhD, Richard S. Crow, MD, Aaron R. Folsom, MD, MPH, Peter J. Hannan, MStat, Duanping Liao, MD, PhD, Cees A. Swenne, PhD, and Evert G. Schouten, MD, PhD, "Clinical Investigation and Reports: Low Heart Rate Variability in a 2-Minute Rhythm Strip Predicts Risk of Coronary Heart Disease and Mortality from Several Causes: The ARIC Study," *Circulation* 102 (2000): 1239–1244.

36 Robert M. Carney, Kenneth E. Freedland, and Richard C. Veith, "Depression, the Autonomic Nervous System, and Coronary Heart Disease," *Psychosomatic Medicine* 67 (May–Jun 2005): S29–S33. Studies of medically well, depressed psychiatric patients have found elevated levels of plasma catecholamines and other markers of altered ANS function compared with controls. Studies of depressed patients with coronary heart disease (CHD) have also uncovered evidence of ANS dysfunction, including elevated heart rate, low heart rate variability, exaggerated heart rate responses to physical stressors, high variability in ventricular repolarization, and low baroreceptor sensitivity. All these indicators of ANS dysfunction have been associated with increased risks of mortality and cardiac morbidity in patients with CHD.

37 M. Malik, P. Barthel, R. Schneider, K. Ulm, and G. Schmidt, "Heart-rate Turbulence after Ventricular Premature Beats as a Predictor of Mortality after Acute Myocardial Infarction," *The Lancet* 353, no. 9162 (Apr 24, 1999): 1390–96.

38 U.S. Department of Health and Human Services, National Center for Health Statistics, "Health, United States 2015: Special Feature on Racial and Ethnic Health Disparities" (accessed June 2016), www.cdc.gov /nchs/hus/.

39 A. B. Kulur, N. Haleagrahara, P. Adhikary, and P. S. Jeganathan, "Effect of Diaphragmatic Breathing on Heart Rate Variability in Ischemic Heart Disease with Diabetes," *Arquivos Brasilieros Cardiologia* 92, no. 6 (Jun 2009): 423–29, 440–47, 457–63.

40 Peter Levine is a leading shock and trauma therapist. He uses verbal techniques, combined with a close observation of the client in terms of subtle changes in their autonomic nervous system, as the client regresses to the time of a traumatic event. He wrote *Waking the Tiger* (Berkeley: North Atlantic Books, 1997). Since then, his teaching has grown into a form called Somatic Experiencing.

41 Stephen Porges developed, patented, and marketed a vagal-tone monitor to measure HRV through a small company called Delta-Biometrics, Inc. That company no longer exists; however, there are now many vagal-tone measuring devices manufactured by other companies.

42 James Oschman, PhD is a research scientist and author of the bestselling book *Energy Medicine* (London: Churchill Livingstone, 2000).

43 The Listening Project Protocol is now available through Integrated Listening Systems as the "Safe and Sounds Protocol: A Portal to Social Engagement," http://integratedlistening.com/ssp-safe-sound-protocol.

44 John T. Cottingham, Stephen W. Porges, and Todd Lyon, "Effects of Soft Tissue Mobilization (Rolfing Pelvic Lift) on Parasympathetic Tone in Two Age Groups," *Physical Therapy* 68, no. 3 (Mar 1988): 352–56.

45 D. Buskila and H. Cohen, "Comorbidity of Fibromyalgia and Psychiatric Disorders," *Current Pain and Headache Reports* 11, no. 5 (Oct 2007): 333–38.

46 P. Schweinhardt, K. M. Sauro, and M. C. Bushnell, "Fibromyalgia: a disorder of the brain?" *Neuroscientist* 14, no. 5 (2008): 415–21.

47 A systematic review of antidepressant efficacy failed to demonstrate superior effectiveness compared to psychotherapy, alternative therapy such as exercise, acupuncture, and relaxation, or active intervention controls such as sham acupuncture or therapies not specific to depression. Arif Khan, Charles Faucett, P. Lichtenberg, I. A. Kirsch, and W. A. Brown, "A Systematic Review of Comparative Efficacy of Treatments and Controls for Depression," *PLOS* (Jul 30, 2012), http://dx.doi.org/10.1371/journal.pone.0041778.

48 My primary biomechanical craniosacral teacher is Alain Gehin, the French osteopath who wrote *The Atlas of Manipulative Techniques for the Cranium and the Face.* (See note 5 above.)

49 Monica J. Fletcher, Jane Upton, Judith Taylor-Fishwick, Sonia A. Buist, Christine Jenkins, John Hutton, Neil Barnes, Thys Van Der Molen, John W. Walsh, Paul Jones, and Samantha Walker, "COPD Uncovered: An International Survey on the Impact of Chronic Obstructive Pulmonary Disease [COPD] on a Working-Age Population," *BMC Public Health Journal* 11, no. 612 (2011), www.biomedcentral .com/1471-2458/11/612#B1, doi :10.1186/1471-2458-11-612.

50 *The 10 Leading Causes of Death in the World, 2000 and 2012,* World Health Organization Fact Sheet No. 310 (Geneva, Switzerland: World Health Organization, 2013).

51 Robert I. Miller and Sterling K. Clarren, "Long-Term Developmental Outcomes in Patients with Deformational Plagiocephaly," *Pediatrics* 105, no. 2 (Feb 2000): e26.

52 David G. Simons, MD, Janet G. Travell, MD, and Lois S. Simons, PT, *Myofascial Pain and Dysfunction: The Trigger Point Manual,* 6th ed., vol. 2 (London: Churchill Livingstone, 2008).

53 Ida P. Rolf, PhD, *Rolfing: Reestablishing the Natural Alignment and Structural Integration of the Human Body for Vitality and Well-Being,* rev. ed. (Rochester, VT: Healing Arts Press, 1989).

54 John T. Cottingham, Stephen W. Porges, and Todd Lyon, "Effects of Soft Tissue Mobilization (Rolfing Pelvic Lift) on Parasympathetic Tone in Two Age Groups," *Physical Therapy* 68, no. 3 (Mar 1988): 352–56. Their experiment is discussed in detail in Chapter 4.

55 C. C. Lunardi, F. A. Marques da Silva, Rodrigues Mendes, Marques A. P. Stelmach, and Fernandes Carvalho, "Is there an Association Between Postural Balance and Pulmonary Function in Adults with Asthma?" *Clinics* 68, no. 11 (São Paulo, Brazil: Department of Physical Therapy, School of Medicine, University of São Paulo, Nov 2013).

56 D. M. Kado, M. H. Huang, H. S. Karlamangla, E. Barrett-Connor, and G.A. Greendale, "Hyperkyphotic Posture Predicts Mortality in Older Community-Dwelling Men and Women: A Prospective Study," *Journal of the American Geriatric Society* 52, no. 10 (Oct 2004): 1662–67.

57 *Mayo Clinic Newsletter* (Nov 3, 2000).

58 Alf Breig, *Adverse Mechanical Tension in the Central Nervous System: An Analysis of Cause and Effect: Relief by Functional Neurosurgery* (Stockholm: Almqvist & Wiksell International, 1978).

59 Roger W. Sperry, "Roger Sperry's Brain Research," *Bulletin of The Theosophy Science Study Group* 26, no. 3–4 (1988): 27–28. Also see Sperry's review of *The Formation of Nerve Connections* by R. M. Gaze in *Quarterly Review of Biology* 46 (Jun 1971): 198.

60 A. I. Kapandji, *The Physiology of the Joints*, 6th ed., vol. 3 (London: Churchill Livingstone, 2008).

61 T. A. Smitherman, R. Burch, H. Sheikh, and E. Loder, "The Prevalence, Impact, and Treatment of Migraine and Severe Headaches in the United States: A Review of Statistics from National Surveillance Studies," *Headache* 53, no. 3 (Mar 7, 2013): 427–36.

62 L. D. Goldberg, "The Cost of Migraine and its Treatment," *American Journal of Managed Care* 11, no. 2 suppl. (Jun 2005): S62–67.

63 David G. Simons, MD, Janet G. Travell, MD, and Lois S. Simons, PT, *Myofascial Pain and Dysfunction: The Trigger Point Manual*, 6th ed., vol. 2 (London: Churchill Livingstone, 2008).

64 M. S. Robbins and R. B. Lipton, "The Epidemiology of Primary Headache Disorders," *Seminal Neurology* 30 (Apr 2010): 107–19.

65 Jes Olesen, *Headaches*, 3rd ed. (Philadelphia: Lippincott, Williams & Wilkins, 2006), 246–47.

66 R. C. Kessler, W. T. Chiu, O. Demler, K. R. Merikangas, and E. E. Walters, "Prevalence, Severity, and Comorbidity of 12-Month DSM-IV Disorders in the National Comorbidity Survey Replication," *Archives of General Psychiatry* 62, no. 6 (Jun 2005): 617–27.

67 Phil Barker, *Psychiatric and Mental Health Nursing: The Craft of Caring* (London: Arnold, 2003).

68 Michael Passer, Ronald Smith, Nigel Holt, Andy Bremner, Ed Sutherland, and Michael Vliek, *Psychology* (UK: McGrath Hill Higher Education, 2009).

69 *The National Intimate Partner and Sexual Violence Survey* (Atlanta, GA: National Center for Injury Prevention and Control, Centers for Disease Control and Prevention, 2017), www.cdc.gov/violenceprevention/nisvs/.

70 M. J. Breiding, J. Chen, and M. C. Black, *Intimate Partner Violence in the United States—2010* (Atlanta, GA: National Center for Injury Prevention and Control, Centers for Disease Control and Prevention, 2014), www.cdc.gov/violenceprevention/pdf/cdc_nisvs_ipv _report_2013_v17_single_a.pdf.

71 T. Frodi, E. Meisenzahl, T. Zetsche, R. Bottlender, C. Born, C. Groll, M. Jäger, G. Leinsinger, K. Hahn, and H.J. Möller, "Enlargement of the Amygdala in Patients with a First Episode of Major Depression," *Biological Psychiatry* 51, no. 9 (May 1, 2002): 708–14.

72 Bruce S. McEwen, "L1 Stress Induced, Hippocampal, Amygdala and Prefrontal Cortex Plasticity and Mood Disorders," *Behavioral Pharmacology* 15, no. 5–6 (2001): A1.

73 There was no published report from this treatment project. This summary is condensed from personal conversations with psychologist Marc Levin over several years.

74 Thomas Insel, "Antidepressants: A Complicated Picture," *The National Institute of Mental Health Directors Blog* (Dec 6, 2011), www.nimh.nih .gov/about/directors/thomas-insel/blog/2011/antidepressants-a -complicated-picture.shtml.

75 Peter Wehrwein, "Astounding Increase in Antidepressant Use by Americans," *Harvard Health Blog* (Oct 20, 2011), www.health .harvard.edu/blog/astounding-increase-in-antidepressant-use-by -americans-201110203624.

76 Andreas Vilhelmsson, "Depression and Antidepressants: A Nordic Perspective," *Frontiers in Public Health* 1, no. 30 (Aug 26, 2013), doi: 10.3389/fpubh.2013.00030.

77 Craig W. Lindsley, ed., "2013 Statistics for Global Prescription Medications," *ACS Chemical Neuroscience* 5, no. 4 (Apr 16, 2014): 250– 251, www.ncbi.nlm.nih.gov/pmc/articles/PMC3990946/, doi: 10.1021 /cn500063v.

78 Jay C. Fournier, MA, Robert J. DeRubeis, PhD, Steven D. Hollon, PhD, Sona Dimidjian, PhD, Jay D. Amsterdam, MD, Richard C. Shelton, MD, and Jan Fawcett, MD, "Antidepressant Drug Effects and Depression Severity: A Patient-Level Meta-analysis," *Journal of the American Medical Association* 303 (2010): 47–53.

79 Mark Olfson, MD and Steven C. Marcus, PhD, "National Patterns in Antidepressant Medication Treatment," *Archives of General Psychiatry* 66, no. 8 (2009): 848–856, doi: 10.1001/archgenpsychiatry.2009.81.

80 R. C. Kessler, P. A. Berglund, O. Demler, R. Jin, K. R. Merikangas, and E.E. Walters, "Lifetime Prevalence and Age-of-Onset Distributions of DSM-IV Disorders in the National Comorbidity Survey Replication," *Archives of General Psychiatry* 62, no. 6 (Jun 2005): 593–602.

81 See Chapter 5, "Relieving COPD and Hiatal Hernia," for more about hiatal hernias and their treatment.

82 Centers for Disease Control and Prevention, "Prevalence of Autism Spectrum Disorder Among Children Aged 8 Years—Autism and Developmental Disabilities Monitoring Network," *Surveillance Summaries* (Mar 28, 2010): 1–21.

83 Centers for Disease Control and Prevention Autism and Developmental Disabilities Monitoring Network Surveillance Year 2010 Principal Investigators, Jon Baio, EdS, corresponding author, "Prevalence of Autism Spectrum Disorder among Children Aged 8 Years—Autism and Developmental Disabilities Monitoring Network, 11 Sites, United States, 2010," *Morbidity and Mortality Weekly Report* 63, no. SS02 (Mar 28, 2014): 1–21.

84 Ariane V. Buescher, MSc; Zuleyha Cidav, PhD, Martin Knapp, PhD, and David S. Mandell, ScD, "Costs of Autism Spectrum Disorders in the United Kingdom and the United States," *Journal of the American Medical Association Pediatrics* 168, no. 8 (Aug 2014): 721–28.

85 Tara A. Lavelle, PhD, Milton C. Weinstein, PhD, Joseph P. Newhouse, PhD, Kerim Munir, MD, MPH, DSc, Karen A. Kuhlthau, PhD, and Lisa A. Prosser, PhD, "Economic Burden of Childhood Autism Spectrum Disorders," *Pediatrics* 133, no. 3 (Mar 1, 2014): e520–29.

86 Nicole Ostrow, "Autism Costs More Than 2 Million Dollars over Patient's Lifetime," *Bloomberg Business* (Jun 10, 2014), www.bloomberg.com/news/articles/2014-06-09/autism-costs-more -than-2-million-over-patient-s-life.

87 Also see Erik Borg and S. Allen Counter, "The Middle-Ear Muscles," *Scientific American* 261, no. 2 (Aug 1989): 74–80.

88 The listening project protocol is now available through Integrated Listening Systems as the "Safe and Sounds Protocol: A Portal to Social Engagement," http://integratedlistening.com/ssp-safe-sound-protocol.

89 Porges, S. W., Macellaio, M., Stanfill, S. D., McCue, K., Lewis, G. F., Harden, E. R., and Heilman, K. J., "Respiratory Sinus Arrhythmia and Auditory Processing in Autism: Modifiable Deficits of an Integrated Social Engagement System?" *International Journal of Psychophysiology* 88, no. 3 (2013): 261–270.

90 Stephen W. Porges, Olga V. Bazhenova, Elgiz Bal, Nancy Carlson, Yevgeniya Sorokin, Keri J. Heilman, Edwin H. Cook, and Gregory F. Lewis, "Reducing Auditory Hypersensitivities in Autism Spectrum Disorder: Preliminary Findings Evaluating the Listening Project Protocol," *Frontiers in Pediatrics* 2, no. 80 (Aug 1, 2014), doi: 10.3389/fped.2014.00080.

91 This is based on conversations with Stephen and his lab assistant, who tested the function of my stapedius muscle on two different visits. See also Erik Borg and S. Allen Counter, "The Middle-Ear Muscles," *Scientific American* 261, no. 2 (Aug 1989): 74–80.

92 R. I. Miller and S. K. Clarren, "Long-Term Developmental Outcomes in Patients with Deformational Plagiocephaly," *Pediatrics* 105, no. 2 (Feb 2000), http://pediatrics.aappublications.org/content/105/2/e26.short.

93 Thomas W. Myers, *Anatomy Trains: Myofascial Meridians for Manual and Movement Therapists,* 3rd ed. (London: Churchill Livingstone, 2014).

94 J. Douglas Bremner, MD, "Neuroimaging Studies in Post-Traumatic Stress Disorder," *Current Psychiatry Reports* 4 (2002): 254–63.

INDEX

ABOUT THE AUTHOR

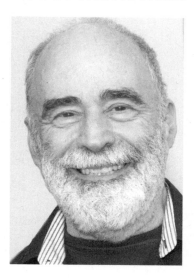

Stanley Rosenberg is an American-born author and body therapist. A Rolfer since 1983 and a practicing craniosacral therapist since 1987, he studied biomechanical craniosacral therapy for many years under Alain Gehin, trained in craniosacral therapy at the Upledger Institute and in biodynamic craniosacral courses with Giorgia Milne, studied applications for treating children with Benjamin Shield, and took courses in osteopathy with Jean-Pierre Barral.

For many years he led a school in Denmark, teaching structural integration, myofascial release, release of scar tissue, biomechanical craniosacral therapy, visceral massage, and biotensegrity. He is the author of four books, published in Denmark: *Nevermore Pain in the Back, Nevermore Stiff Neck, Pain Relief with Osteomassage,* and *Hwa Yu Tai Chi.* In addition to his work as a body therapist, he has worked in theater— training actors in yoga, acrobatics, and voice—at various institutions, including Yale University, Brandeis University, Swarthmore College, and the National Theatre Schools of Denmark and Iceland. More information about the techniques presented in this book can be found on his website: www.stanleyrosenberg.com.

About North Atlantic Books

North Atlantic Books (NAB) is an independent, nonprofit publisher committed to a bold exploration of the relationships between mind, body, spirit, and nature. Founded in 1974, NAB aims to nurture a holistic view of the arts, sciences, humanities, and healing. To make a donation or to learn more about our books, authors, events, and newsletter, please visit www.northatlanticbooks.com.

North Atlantic Books is the publishing arm of the Society for the Study of Native Arts and Sciences, a 501(c)(3) nonprofit educational organization that promotes cross-cultural perspectives linking scientific, social, and artistic fields. To learn how you can support us, please visit our website.